Microcosms of the brain

what sensorimotor systems reveal about the mind

Douglas Tweed

Professor, Departments of Physiology and Medicine, University of Toronto, Canada

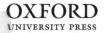

OXFORD
UNIVERSITY PRESS

OXFORD
UNIVERSITY PRESS

Great Clarendon Street, Oxford OX2 6DP

Oxford University Press is a department of the University of Oxford.
It furthers the University's objective of excellence in research, scholarship,
and education by publishing worldwide in

Oxford New York

Auckland Bangkok Buenos Aires Cape Town Chennai
Dar es Salaam Delhi Hong Kong Istanbul Karachi Kolkata
Kuala Lumpur Madrid Melbourne Mexico City Mumbai Nairobi
São Paulo Shanghai Taipei Tokyo Toronto

Oxford is a registered trade mark of Oxford University Press
in the UK and in certain other countries

Published in the United States
by Oxford University Press Inc., New York

British Library Cataloguing in Publication Data

Data available

ISBN 0 19 850735 6 (hardback)
0 19 852893 0 (paperback)

10 9 8 7 6 5 4 3 2 1

Typeset by Integra Software Services Pvt. Ltd., Pondicherry, India
Printed in Great Britain
on acid-free paper by Biddles Ltd., Guilford & King's Lynn

To my parents

Acknowledgements

Novelists sometimes take their titles from fragments of poetry. In a similar way, I have taken mine from a phrase of the neurophysiologist Roger Carpenter, who wrote that the neuronal system that controls our eyes constitutes 'a microcosm of the brain', meaning that the system is relatively simple yet incorporates many aspects of brain function in general. Here I pursue the theme that microcosms like this one provide an arena where the fundamental principles of brain function can be identified.

I have tried to present this view in a way that is clear to readers outside neuroscience. For their feedback on my earlier attempts to do this, I thank the students in my introductory courses at the University of Western Ontario and the University of Toronto.

For their comments on the manuscript I thank Karl Beykirch, Dianne Broussard, Alina Constantin, Douglas Crawford, Buzz Currie, Susanne Ferber, Caroline Härdter, Thomas Haslwanter, Cynthia Hawkins, Denise Henriques, Julio Martinez-Trujillo, Pieter Medendorp, Hubert Misslisch, Matthias Niemeier, Kai Schreiber, James Sharpe, Mike Smith, Dave Tomlinson, Arnold, Glenyce and Dean Tweed, Erik Viirre and Tutis Vilis. I am grateful also to Caroline Härdter for preparing the index and to Danitza Goche Montes for secretarial assistance.

I thank Vanessa Whitting, formerly of Oxford University Press, for inviting me to write this book, and Martin Baum, Kate Martin and the copy editors and graphic artists at OUP for their agreeability and attention in seeing the project through. For their support during the writing and earlier development of the book I am grateful to the Canadian Institutes of Health Research, the University of Toronto, the University of Western Ontario, the University of Tübingen, and the Deutsche Forschungsgemeinschaft.

Contents

Chapter 1

Brain of darkness

Present-day knowledge of the brain resembles in some ways earlier Europeans' knowledge of Africa. Explorers have mapped the coastline in detail, but the interior is mostly uncharted. We know a lot about the input side of the brain, where our sense organs gather information and transmit it centrally. And we understand almost as much about the output side, where commands emerge from the center to activate our muscles. But everything in between, the whole machinery of sensorimotor transformation that converts our sensations and stored knowledge into purposeful action, is more mysterious. Anatomists have brought back reports about the wiring of nuclei and cortices throughout the brain, but still we know little about what these structures are doing. Until we find out, our functional map of the interior will remain mostly a blank page, enlivened with fanciful images. Penetrating the interior, I believe, will require techniques beyond those that have served us on the peripheries. My aim in this book is to present one promising approach, laying out its logic and describing some of its early successes.

The main barrier to progress is the sheer complexity of the brain. In daily life of course we rarely notice how intricate are our own inner workings. We sense our surroundings with little conscious effort. Except when we are trying to rumba, we seem to move our bodies with ease. We think nothing of navigating a room without hitting the walls or furniture. Our feeling of effortlessness makes this sort of purposeful action seem simple, but the feeling is deceptive. Beneath the level of consciousness, prodigious control systems are at work. Every movement of our eyes, for instance, is powered by twelve small muscles, six per eyeball, steered by some 60 000 nerve cells, called motor neurons, in the brainstem.[1] All these neurons are themselves complex structures. Stained black with silver salts and viewed under a microscope they look like bare trees in winter, with hundreds of branching limbs, every twig a powerful information processor in its own right. And these 60 000 motor neurons are merely one output path for the 100 billion neurons of the central nervous system.[2] Neuroscientists recite statistics like these with a certain pride, but there is an urgent problem here. To paraphrase Oscar Wilde, how can I hope to understand a system of this complexity when I am baffled by my manual can opener? What *sort* of understanding can I expect? What questions can I answer? In this book I will develop the idea that the brain is comprehensible, in a certain rigorous sense, if we approach it with the right questions.

I will argue for a threefold path through the functional interior of the brain. First, I will suggest that we begin by studying not whole human brains but simpler neural systems—maybe surprisingly simple ones. I will argue that the ground principles of intelligent, purposeful behavior will be clearest in small subsystems of the human brain, operating largely below the level of consciousness. Second, I will suggest that most of our knowledge of the brain will have to be stored and manipulated inside computers. It is simply beyond us to cope with the complexity of even the humblest brain circuits without electronic help. Neuroscientists of the future will rely more and more on simulations to draw out the consequences of their theories, as physicists do now in exploring the complexities of weather, aerodynamics, and galactic collisions. And third, to be able to write these simulations, we will have to seek out patterns or ordering principles in the brain, something corresponding to the natural laws that underlie physicists' simulations.

Simple minds

Being complex is better than the alternative. If we had simpler brains we would be even worse equipped to understand them. Houseflies, with about a milligram of brain apiece, have minds perhaps a million times simpler than ours, and it is hard to believe that they have a deeper insight into their own psyches.

But if we can't currently understand ourselves, and flies can't understand themselves, still *we* might be able to understand *them*. Later, the lessons we learned from the fly brain might help us analyze our own. That is the idea behind a distinguished line of experiments that have shown how signals from an insect's compound eyes control its flight path, adjust its attitude, extend its landing gear, and so on. Another approach, and the main one I will pursue in this book, is to study human brains right from the start but to begin with simple subsystems of them. Either way, the idea is to seek out general principles in some setting where we aren't overwhelmed. Just as physicists begin with manageable objects like particles, pendulums, and frictionless planes, building up slowly to more complex cases, we begin with little pieces of brain and work from there.

A drawback to studying human subsystems, as opposed to whole flies, is that a fly brain is pretty much an autonomous, self-contained data processor which can be studied in isolation, whereas any subsystem of the human brain is part of a larger whole, constantly influenced by other centers. But the human approach has compensating advantages. Most importantly, we have inside information. When we try to figure out how a human brain works, we can draw on our own years of experience as living humans. This sort of intuition is incomplete and sometimes misleading, but I will argue that it is nevertheless one of the best guides we have through the complexity of the brain. It can even help us understand distantly related creatures like flies, though it is most useful with people. Another advantage of studying human subsystems is that it puts us on a staircase—a long staircase but an unbroken one—from simple circuits up to our ultimate goal, the whole human brain. By expanding our subsystem of interest to incorporate more and more of the networks that interact with it, we can gradually make our way toward a full brain model.

Arguably the best subsystems to start with are not the very simplest ones like the knee jerk or the pupillary light reflex, but systems of intermediate complexity. Our systems should be simple enough to be manageable but complex enough to show many features of the brain at large, features like learning, dynamics, feedback guidance, and multisensory inference. In this book I will draw my illustrations from several such systems of intermediate complexity, including visual processors and control systems for the eye, head, and arm.

It's the motion

Ideally we should study circuitry that receives some sort of sensory input and uses that information to control some action, moving the eyes for instance, or the head, tongue, or limbs. In other words, the system should perform a sensorimotor transformation. I think this is important because sensorimotor transformation is what the brain is for. Its whole uncharted middle is given over to sensorimotor tasks, converting sight and sound and other sensory data into purposeful motion.

That is its only job. Our senses, thoughts, and emotions exist only to guide our action, though it is easy to forget this fact. It can seem as though the function of vision is to cast pictures in our heads, but this isn't so. Our brains were built by natural selection,[3] and natural selection doesn't care about pictures in our heads unless they make a difference to our genetic success, which usually means a difference in our motor behavior. Wishes, fears, appetites, and all our other attitudes and emotions exist to influence our actions. There is no point perceiving food, danger, or a friend unless the perception activates an appropriate motor program. It is no coincidence that organisms that don't move much, like trees and mushrooms, don't have much of a brain. (At the other end of the spectrum, humans are the world's most versatile movers. Flies fly and land, feed and mate, and rub their hands together; horses trot, canter, and gallop; but humans speak, gesture, juggle, swim, play the trombone, rumba, turn cartwheels, throw, pole vault, and handle thousands of tools.)

Are there any brain systems that aren't ultimately concerned with motor control? The brain does perform jobs that aren't usually called sensorimotor.

Its autonomic circuits, for instance, control hormone levels, blood pressure, and so on. But these tasks differ in no essential way from sensorimotor transformations. Their sensory inputs and data processing may be entirely unconscious rather than partly available to consciousness, and their motor outputs may involve glands or smooth muscles rather than skeletal muscles, but they work on the same principles as the sensorimotor transformations that I will discuss in this book. In what follows, I will use the term sensorimotor to cover autonomic systems as well.

When neural systems appear especially inscrutable or 'human' we may call them cognitive, but still they were shaped for just one purpose: to control our motor action. Of course large parts of the brain are concerned not with immediate, on-line control of action, but with accumulating wisdom. Our brains gather and store reams of data about how the world works, whether red means stop or go, whether socks go with sandals, and so on. Ultimately, though, the sole purpose of all this stored information is to promote our genetic success by driving appropriate motor activity. Not that every piece of stored wisdom really will contribute to genetic success. I have neurons dedicated to holding the information, 'Tell y'all a story 'bout a man named Jed. Poor mountain man barely kept his family fed.'[4] Knowing this theme song hasn't yet aided my reproductive success, but the point is, you never know. Natural selection has designed us to gather information voraciously because it is hard to predict what knowledge will come in handy.

It was motor performance, almost alone, that drove the evolution of the brain. Organisms whose motor activity led to reproductive success passed their genes to the next generation. In this way the brain was shaped from the outside in, or better, from the motor periphery all the way back to the sensors. Ultimately, it was motor performance that shaped even the lens of the eye. All the brain's inner workings, all its thoughts and feelings, membranes and synapses, neurotransmitters and receptors, are there only to achieve the right relation between sensory input and motor output. It was by weighing sensorimotor transformations one against another that natural selection made us what we are. At bottom, a human personality is a phenomenally complex, interlocking system of sensorimotor transformations.

The mysteries

This point can be pressed further. It can be argued that sensorimotor transformations are the key to understanding all aspects of brain function, including the supposedly mysterious ones like conscious thought. This thesis was presented forcefully by the brilliant British mathematician Alan Turing in a paper in 1950.[5] I agree with Turing and his followers that our conscious inner life, our vivid sensorium, our emotions and intentions, are aspects of our sensorimotor transformations experienced from the inside. Consciousness is what it is like to be a sensorimotor organism. I think this view is winning acceptance, that mind is order and information, not ectoplasm or a brew of chemicals, and—though this is somewhat further from general consent—that all the information that matters for consciousness and personal identity is that which influences our sensorimotor performance. I see it as a healthy sign that most science fiction treats androids as conscious (though many science-fiction shows on TV also imply that the galaxy is full of attractive, English-speaking aliens in snug outfits, so philosophers wouldn't find this argument conclusive).

Some people disagree with Turing. They think that our inner mental life must be separable from sensorimotor performance. They think that it would be possible for an android to match human behavior in all details, including the way that our behavior changes with learning, and yet be unconscious. They doubt that outer space is filled with Lycra-clad humanoids. Since 1950, the arguments for and against Turing's view have been presented at length. I confess that I have regarded this issue as settled since I was converted, years ago, from mind–body dualism to my current views, partly by the writings of Turing, W.V. Quine, and Hilary Putnam. If you are skeptical you can read this book as an account of neural performance with no bearing on consciousness. The philosophical debate you can follow elsewhere. But the debate over consciousness shouldn't obscure the straightforward point, which is a guiding thesis in this book, that natural selection had only motor performance to go on in shaping the brain.

The threefold path

One of my aims in this book is to lay out a set of fundamental concepts, one per chapter, that I think we need in order to understand the workings of the brain. In this chapter I have discussed the primacy of motor performance in directing the brain's evolution. In the next ten chapters I will introduce *optimization, computation, complexity, learning, dynamics, interfaces, loops, degrees of freedom, information,* and *inference.* In textbooks these topics are explained mathematically. Here I try to lay out the issues as far as possible without equations. I have always found that even the most intimidating mathematical proofs are essentially simple ideas worked out in hair-raising detail. They are daunting mainly because of the bookkeeping aspect, not because of the underlying concepts. If you are interested in the details, I provide references to further readings. But here I will illustrate the ten concepts using simple sensorimotor examples. I chose my illustrations not because they provide a survey of current research or because they are all among the most important discoveries in the field. I chose them because they are the clearest examples I know.

Why these ten concepts and not more obviously psychological ones like consciousness, emotions, attention, semantics, and so on? The ten are more fundamental. They are also much less vague: each of them is the subject of a rigorous mathematical theory, though in some cases the theories are still in development. I will argue that these concepts can help provide a basis for the computerized neuroscience of the future.

In the first five chapters I lay out a program—I suggest a viewpoint and a set of questions that I hope will be useful for neuroscience. There is a precedent for this sort of thing in the research programs of mathematics and physics, for instance in Felix Klein's *Erlangen* program, where he suggested that vast realms of exotic geometry could be studied and unified by exploring symmetries. Or the modern program for nonlinear dynamics, where complex, high-dimensional systems are rendered manageable by focusing on what are called their singularities. Here I will suggest that complex, high-dimensional neural systems can be rendered comprehensible by focusing on their optimization principles.

A developing theme will be that the last seven concepts, all those after *complexity* in the list, can be subsumed as aspects of optimization. Learning, for instance, is nothing more than the brain optimizing itself. And a brain that self-optimizes can automatically learn to cope with dynamics and interfaces, to handle loops, to coordinate its degrees of freedom, and so on. As we proceed, then, the approach we are taking will resolve into the threefold path: we will work with sensorimotor systems, starting with simpler ones; we will leave the details to computers; and we will let optimization be our guide.

Chapter 2

Guide to the interior

In unknown territory a good guide is indispensable, and a bad one can be disastrous. But 'good' doesn't have to mean 'infallible'; a guide that occasionally errs may be helpful all the same. I will discuss this idea as a methodological precept for neuroscience, but it is interesting to observe, as evidence of its validity, that the same precept was discovered long ago by the sensory systems in the brain itself, all of which rely on guiding assumptions or rules of thumb that are usually correct but sometimes mislead. Consider hearing. A stereo recording played through headphones can give you a vivid impression of sounds coming from points in your head or in space remote from the real speakers in your ears. In other words your brain is fooled into hearing things that aren't there. Why does it fall for this? The headphones project into your two ears sound sequences that are similar but not identical. Your brain interprets the differences in loudness and timing as clues to the locations of the sound sources, which is reasonable because these differences usually do reflect source location. Your unconscious assumption that binaural disparity reflects geometry is what allows you to pinpoint sounds. If you didn't make this assumption, you would be immune to deception by headphones, but the price you would pay would be your spatial hearing. Every sensory system relies on this sort of useful but imperfect assumption. Many optical illusions, for instance, arise when a picture violates some usually sound interpretive principle built into the brain. Without these principles, we would be almost helpless to interpret sensory signals.

A similar situation faces us when we study the brain. We need guiding principles to help us interpret the data. A good guide, meaning a principle that is based on some valid generalization about the brain, even if it occasionally misleads, can help us to insights that we would otherwise never attain. A bad guide, based on a preconception or overgeneralization, can lead us into quagmires of error. I discuss one false guide, linearity, in the final section of Chapter 3. In the present chapter I will defend one guiding principle that I consider indispensable to neuroscience, namely optimization.

The optimized brain

If you want to understand a complex biological system like the brain, the most useful working assumption you can make is that it is optimally designed for some purpose. Probably this has always been the main source of insight in biology, but until recently it was considered gauche, in certain circles, to say so in public. Any talk of purpose or design was called teleology, which was seen as a philosophical error, most likely because it was thought to imply a conscious designer or some sort of backward causation, where modern organisms shaped their own evolution. But purpose and design have since been cleared of these charges. It is now understood that biological purpose and design can arise from the known laws of physics through Darwin's process of natural selection, or 'survival of the

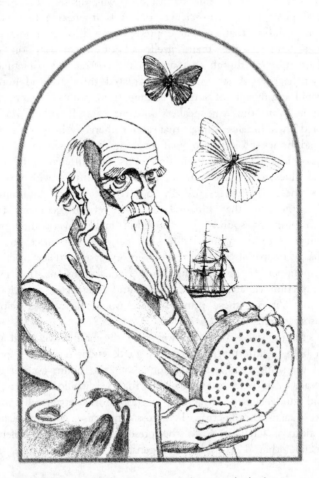

Fig. 2.1 Darwin with the sieve, representing natural selection.

fittest'.[6, 7] Over millions of generations natural selection sifts through the gene pool, weeding out the bad genes, promoting the good ones, gradually nudging its creatures toward optimality. The same process underlies a mathematical technique called the genetic algorithm, which is used to solve optimization problems in science and industry. Faced, then, with a poorly understood organ or system, we know how to proceed. If we can identify the system's function and work out the optimal design for that function, then we have at least a rough idea of what to look for in the actual design. This optimization approach has been successfully applied to topics throughout biology, from frog jumping to honeycomb architecture to the human brain.

It may seem optimistic, or delusional, to apply the word *optimized* to the human brain. If our brains are so optimized, why do people smoke, or get abducted by aliens? Why did I buy those stretch pants? Why did a friend of my uncle's once slam a kitchen drawer on his own pendulous gut? These are important questions, but they don't really touch the optimization issue. Optimized doesn't mean brilliant, it means doing certain things as well as they can be done given various constraints, and that is entirely consistent with occasionally slamming a drawer on your own belly. That we are often pretty dim doesn't mean that our brains aren't optimized in all sorts of important ways.

Genetic space

It is helpful to regard natural selection as unfolding in genetic space, which is an abstract realm where every point represents a genome. Every genome possesses a certain level of fitness, though that level isn't fixed through time. As climate or customs change, or as new diseases, predators, or prey appear, a genome that was formerly viable may become passé. But this flux doesn't alter the fact that natural selection is an optimizing process, moving through genetic space in the current direction of increasing fitness.

Limits to optimization

Like most optimizing processes, natural selection often—probably almost always—gets stuck in local optima rather than in the global optimum. It settles, that is, for some good design rather than finding the very best design. One clue that this has happened to us is that our eyeballs are wired inside out. In the retina, which is the thin, light-sensitive sheet covering the interior back surface of the eye, the photoreceptor cells—the rods and cones—point back toward the rear wall of the eye rather than forward toward the light. Wiring them the right way round, as they are in the eyes of octopuses, would give us better vision, but some early turn in our evolution must have carried us off the path to octopus eyes.

Even if an organ is evolving toward an optimal design it may not have had time to get there. An example may be the human spine. Many people have back problems, and the reason is that our spines are poorly constructed for upright walkers like us. Engineers claim that they could design a better support, presumably some sort of column running up the center of the torso rather than the back, with radial shelves to hold our internal organs. So why have we been saddled with these second-rate spinal columns? The reason is that we inherited them from our ancestors, who walked around on all fours. For them, the spine was a horizontal beam, supporting their internal organs like a clothes line holding laundry, and for this purpose it was well designed. Only when we reared up on our hind legs did the design become less satisfactory. Since then, it has at least partly adapted to its new job; the lumbar vertebrae, for instance, have grown wider and thicker to support the tower above them. Given enough millennia, the design may improve further, maybe moving toward the engineers' optimum. On the other hand, an organ may never reach optimality if some imperfect design turns out to be good enough or if the environment and therefore the demands on the system change faster than evolution can catch up.

Occasionally natural selection may worsen the design of its creatures. It may promote 'rogue genes' which hamper or kill their carriers. Or it may favor one species over another whose members are in some sense fitter: in one species, every single member may be exquisitely specialized for swamp life, but if the swamp dries up, that species may perish while another survives because it is more diversified. Or luckier. Chance plays a role in evolution, as it does also in many optimization algorithms that run on computers. A mutation that could lead to a better design may not happen to appear. Or it may show up in an individual, but a boulder crushes the glorious mutant before it can procreate. On the whole, though, natural selection tends to improve the design of its organisms.

Knowing what's good for you

A separate issue is that we may have trouble recognizing what is being optimized. Natural selection preserved the gene for sickle-cell anemia, despite its dire effects, because it protects against malaria, but figuring that out took some insight because the functional advantages of sickle cells aren't obvious at first glance. There are probably many similar instances where functional advantages aren't immediately obvious, or involve compromises among many factors. A famous case is the Irish elk, which became extinct about 10 000 years ago.[8] It was the biggest deer that ever lived, but big as it was, it had disproportionately large antlers, weighing up to 40 kg and stretching as much as $3\frac{1}{2}$ m across—probably about twice the span of your outstretched arms. Early in the twentieth century biologists were baffled by the big horns. Surely such huge antlers had no practical use, so why did natural selection produce them? Some scientists even felt that the Irish elk died out precisely because of its huge antlers. Tangled up in branches, stuck in elevators, it perished, according to this view, because of

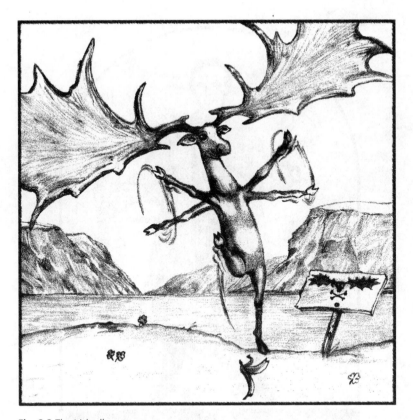

Fig. 2.2 The Irish elk.

its cumbersome headgear. Nowadays, we think the antlers served in sexual display or ritualized combat,[8] but in any case the point is that the purpose of a feature may be hard to discern.

Another problem is that natural selection is looking for optimal loci in genetic space—the set of all possible genomes—and many of us have a poorly developed intuition for genetic space. A design that seems to us optimal for some purpose may simply be unachievable by any genome. Many useful features, such as x-ray vision, may be unattainable because no genomes anywhere in genetic space give rise to them.

So natural selection is slow and subject to chance, it gets stuck in local optima, and often we need some ingenuity to work out what is being optimized. Should we give up in disgust, or are these just minor pitfalls to watch out for? In practice, it is remarkable how little a problem they are. All we have to do is keep in mind that organisms are seldom stable in a global optimum. They tend to be *en route* to a local optimum. Even if the brain is far from optimal in some respect, our efforts to deduce the optimal design help us to understand the task, and they lead us to meaningful tests of our theories: can the optimal design do something that our current

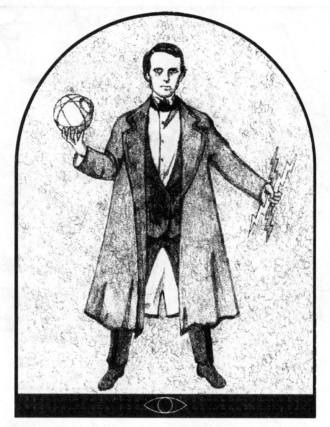

Fig. 2.3 Hermann von Helmholtz contributed to electromagnetic theory and sensorimotor science.

model can't? How does the brain perform on the same test? To me, abjuring optimization methods on the grounds that natural selection isn't a perfect optimizer seems like covering our ears and eyes because they are sometimes fooled by illusions. Optimization is a flawed guide, but it is the best one we have to the dark places of the brain. It is almost the only way to explain not just how we are built, but why we are built that way. From the pioneering work of Hermann von Helmholtz in the 19th century until the present, as I will show in later chapters, no other approach to the brain has yielded so many significant and correct predictions.

The lawnmower problem

There is a school of neuroscientists that tries to make a go of exploring the brain without guides. They eschew speculation, proud that their models contain nothing beyond the currently available data. They posit no neurons, no connections, no membrane or synaptic properties beyond those that have been documented in the brain. They believe that this policy keeps them in contact with reality, but it can have the reverse effect. The problem is that the brain is a jungle, and we know next to nothing about what is going on in there. Of all the cell types involved in a given brain system, how many do we know about right now, and how many remain to be discovered? Considering just the neurons we have identified already, how well do we know them? How thoroughly have we explored their behavior under the full range of conditions they face in life? Surely it is optimistic to think that we have, say, ten per cent of the relevant information about the parts of the system and their interaction.

We are like a person who orders a lawnmower that has to be assembled from the shipped components, but then finds that the box, when it arrives, is broken and contains only ten per cent of the parts. We can doggedly restrict ourselves to the available pieces, and then proudly announce that the assembled contraption uses only parts found in the box, but it won't look much like the lawnmower we ordered, and likely it won't cut grass. If we are handy enough, we would do better to deduce what parts are missing and replace them with home-made pieces. We may be wrong in many details—the colors, the materials, even the precise shapes of the missing bits—but the results are likely to be better than the ten per cent solution.

Similar problems face scientists who reconstruct artefacts and organisms dug out of the clay. If we come across a tyrannosaurus skeleton we may not find her femurs or her quadriceps, but we know something must have joined her hips with her knees and extended her legs, or she would have fallen over. In other words, judgements about function guide us when we reconstruct dinosaurs. Likewise for the lawnmower. And likewise, I suggest, for the brain, where a knowledge of sensorimotor purpose is crucial in allowing us to fill in pieces that haven't yet been found. An excessively sober approach that restricts us to known anatomy will yield brain models about as valuable as the ten per cent lawnmower.

The available information is scantier for the brain than for dinosaur skeletons, but that only increases the need for judicious reconstruction. The fewer pieces we have in hand, the more we have to derive by clever guesses. If we rebuild a fossil from a single mandible we will have plenty of scope for error, but almost anything we come up with will be more plausible than the sober, conservative solution of using only the available fossil, reconstructing the creature as a free-living jawbone. Experimental tests of the reconstruction are the next step. But without the reconstructions, we won't know what to test, and we won't recognize crucial pieces of the lawnmower when we find them.

Chapter 3

On the shoulders of computers

The dream of creating an artificial mind goes back at least to Rabbi Loewe, who lived in Prague in the 16th century. According to legend, the rabbi fashioned a human-shaped statue called a golem out of the mud of the Moldau river and animated it with a sort of software in the form of a text written in Hebrew on a slip of paper inserted under the creature's tongue.[9] Another pioneer in this field was Dr Frankenstein, but he assembled his creature from prefabricated parts dug out of graveyards, which is cheating. Rabbi Loewe's closest modern successors may be the roboticists, who build their creations out of metal and electronic parts. Brain theorists pursue the same dream in a slightly different way, building our artificial minds inside computer simulations instead of in hardware. This is mainly a matter of convenience. When we want to try out a new idea, we reach for a computer keyboard and mouse, not a blow torch and safety glasses. Development goes faster, and if our creation turns evil and runs amok, we switch off the computer rather than hunting down the creature through the sewers of Prague, as Rabbi Loewe had to do.

Why simulate the brain? We already have a method of creating new minds, by sexual reproduction, so why do we need a new one? A major attraction of the Loewe–Frankenstein project is control. We want the power, not just to turn out new minds but to specify the details, so that, ultimately, we can repair and improve the minds we have. To put this in slightly more sober terms, one goal of brain simulation is to lay the groundwork for neural prostheses.

Unfortunately, prospects appear dim for prostheses in the brain's functional interior. At the sensory periphery they may be helpful—already the cochlear implant has in some cases restored useful hearing to the deaf. But even on the periphery neural prostheses have run into trouble, in part because attempts to link them with the brain have caused epilepsy by a process called kindling. For this and other reasons, I expect we will be able to build a complete artificial brain before we can build, say, an artificial thalamus that interfaces with the rest of a natural brain. And before we learn to build artificial brains or brain parts electronically, we will learn to grow them by genetic engineering. But prostheses aren't the main rationale for trying to simulate the interior.

A better reason for simulating the brain is to test our understanding. Simulations force us to purge our theories of all gaps and vagueness. For a theory, simulation is a test for logical holes, like squeezing an inner tube under water. To build brains inside a computer, we have to analyze them down to a small set of logical concepts: identity, loops, and the logical truth functions such as *not*, *if*, and *or*. If we can do this, we have passed the ultimate test of understanding, by building a mind out of pieces of pure logic.

But the main reason for simulating the brain is that we have no choice. Only by relying on computers can we hope to understand the mind's complexity. Before arguing that brain simulations are necessary, though, I have to discuss whether they are even possible.

Rage against the machine

Some people believe that any plan to simulate the brain is as fanciful as the legend of Rabbi Loewe, because the brain just isn't the sort of thing that can be captured in a computer. The brain, they say, is not a machine. But these skeptics fall into two groups that use the word 'machine' in quite different ways.

Vitalists

Vitalists believe that the laws of physics aren't enough to explain life, but that another force is needed, a 'vital force' that is in some sense non-physical. Officially, vitalism was overthrown by mechanism early in the 20th century, but it still has its quiet adherents, and their last bastion is in the brain. People who accept that the rest of life runs entirely on physics and chemistry can still balk at the mind. Their brand of vitalism, restricted to the brain, is also called mind–body dualism. I suspect that the main force behind any type of vitalism is the simple, raw conviction that life, or thoughts and feelings, just can't be part of any mere mechanism. This conviction may not yield to any brief argument—in my own case, it crumbled over the years as I tried in vain to justify it—but a few remarks may sway less committed vitalists.

Some vitalists are people who dislike being called machines. Maybe they associate the word with tractors and toasters and vacuum cleaners, objects they feel to be below them. Humans are 'a little lower than the angels', but augers and electric toothbrushes are felt to be quite a bit lower still. The assumption is that no machine, however beautiful, intricate, and adaptable, can ever have much moral worth, so if you accepted that humans are machines, you would be obliged to lower your opinion of humanity.

But no logic compels you to do this if you don't want to. If you think that some entity A is glorious whereas some other entity B is shabby, and then you discover that A and B are one and the same, you are not obliged to lower your estimate of A. You could equally well raise your estimate of B. For that matter you might come to value the multifaceted entity A/B even more than you valued A, thanks to the appreciation that your new understanding has brought you. I think this last version is what usually happens among neuroscientists. No one can study the brain without being overcome, again and again, by its wondrous, adaptive complexity. Anyone can prize human qualities like creativity, loyalty, and courage, but it takes a neuroscientist or a roboticist to admire lesser human and animal gifts like our ability to walk across a room without bumping into things.

It is worth mentioning, too, that we can simulate in computers things that are not themselves machines in any normal sense. Using the equations of hydrodynamics, we can simulate a rushing river. So if you don't want the brain to be a machine but you are happy with it being a dynamic system like a river or a thunderstorm or a pulsing force field, then you should have no qualms about simulation.

Distaste for simulation may reflect the idea that a mind that can't be simulated is more mysterious, and mystery is good because understanding things drains all the charm out of them. Alluding to his disintegrating marriage, Charles Ryder in *Brideshead Revisited* says he learned 'the routine and mechanism of her charm . . . She was stripped of all enchantment now'.[10] But this attitude, that understanding kills beauty, is incompatible with science because it encourages obtuseness. For scientists, understanding a thing deepens its charm, unless we learn that it really is disgusting.

A fundamental problem with vitalism is that it is hard even to formulate clearly. What does it mean to say that the forces of life or mind are 'non-physical'? If tomorrow we discovered some new, fundamental aspect of nature, what tests would we apply to decide whether it was physical or non-physical? It is like trying to distinguish technology from magic. The distinction is unclear.

Vitalism may reflect skepticism about the scope of mathematical explanations. Friends of mine who are unmoved by what John Banville calls the 'cold, grave music of mathematics'[11] have told me that math is too limited, too dry and lifeless to capture anything as fluid and dynamic as the mind. That fluid dynamics is a branch of math is not considered a persuasive rejoinder.

Time will tell what mathematical brain theory achieves, but it is safe to say that any aspect of the mind that is beyond the reach of mathematics will also defy explanation by any other means. This is a safe prediction because math expands to swallow new problems, and because there is no great difference between mathematical and other kinds of thinking, except that math makes heavier use of analogy. Generations of mathematicians have defined and studied things like numbers, vectors, linear operators, groups, rings, metrics, manifolds, and so on, all of which are useful in science because they resemble things in the real world. If I am studying a part of nature and I discover that it fits the defining conditions of, say, a vector space, then suddenly I know a great deal more about it; I know all the theorems about vector spaces established by previous generations of mathematicians. The process is no different from the analogizing that goes on all the time in non-mathematical reasoning, except that it is more rigorous and more daring.

Mathematics liberates the imagination. Once you have learned a few techniques for manipulating vectors and surfaces in three-dimensional space, for instance, it is usually a simple matter to extend the same techniques to deal with hyperdimensional, or even infinite-dimensional, spaces, where your unaided intuition can't take you. These techniques apply to all sorts of things that aren't obviously geometric at all. Processes as diverse as thermodynamics, evolution, and learning can be represented as shapes in abstract, hyperdimensional spaces, though intuitively you wouldn't recognize them as being in any way spatial. Mathematics, by expressing everyday things like space in a strange notation, defamiliarizes them. It removes them from under the cover of our preconceptions, allowing us to see analogies and possibilities that are hidden to common sense. The crystal spheres and motive angels of pre-mathematical cosmologies are quaintly familiar inventions compared with the curved space-time and quantum strangeness of mathematical physics.

Mathematical neuroscience, by the way, used to be called *cybernetics* until that word was usurped by science fiction and the Internet. I had hoped it might be restored to respectability, because I like introducing myself as a cyberneticist, but I gave up that dream the day I came across the *Super Cyber Samurai Squad* on TV. Newer names for the field are *information-processing*, *control-systems* or *computational* neuroscience. The last name is the most popular, but it brings us up against the second group of skeptics of brain simulation.

Non-computationalists

These people usually have a high regard for mathematics, but they know that some mathematical operations are forever beyond the reach of any computer, or in other words any machine, though these aren't machines in the loose, everyday sense of the word. Instead they fit a precise definition developed in the 1930s by several scientists, most notably Alan Turing, the brilliant British mathematician mentioned in the previous chapter, who was also a pioneer of computer science (and built computers for his work, during the Second World War, on Britain's secret Bletchley Park project that cracked the German Enigma code). Turing machines, which are part of the foundations of modern computer science, are imaginary devices, idealized supercomputers which Turing devised to explore the essence of computation and thought.

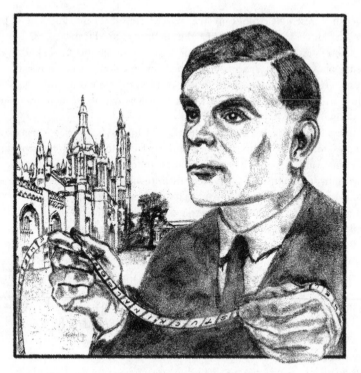

Fig. 3.1 Alan Turing, pioneer of computation theory.

A Turing machine processes data by applying an instruction list, which is a sort of hard-wired program. There is no limit to the amount of data the machine can handle; at any one moment it can hold only a finite set, but the potential size of that set is unbounded, so in this sense the machine has an infinite memory capacity. Similarly, there is no limit to the size of the hard-wired programs Turing machines can run, though any given program must have some finite length. These programs can be written out using the standard elements of computer code: instructions to alter specific data in memory, from 0 to 1 or 1 to 0; the logical truth functions *and, or, not, if-then* and so on; tests for identity as in *if n = 1 then*; and loops, such as *repeat until n = 100*. These machines turn out to be versatile: given any question that can be answered by a digital computer, there is always some Turing machine that can answer it as well.

Turing proved, though, that some tasks are beyond even these universal computers: there are mathematical questions that no Turing machine, and therefore no digital computer, can ever answer. In this regard, a crucial feature of the machines is their finitude: they handle finite (though arbitrarily large) data sets, they run finite programs, and if they deliver an answer at all (rather than getting stuck in an endless loop) their computations consist of finite series of steps. If they could roar through an infinity of steps in

finite time, they could answer new questions, but Turing considered finitude an inescapable feature of computation.

He saw it also as a central feature of the human mind. Turing intended
his machines as models of the mind, and conjectured that they could
answer any question that could ever be answered, in principle, by human
thought. This is the controversial part of his theory. Several authors have
disagreed with him, arguing that human beings can solve puzzles that
Turing machines can't, and that human brains must therefore transcend any
Turing machine. After being apparently demolished by writers like Douglas
Hofstadter[12] in the early 1980s, this argument was revived by the mathematician and physicist Roger Penrose in his 1989 book *The Emperor's New
Mind*.[13] The liner notes to my copy of one of Penrose's books say that he
regards human beings as 'near-miraculous beings', presumably because they
transcend machinehood. But remember that we are talking about Turing
machines here, and there are plenty of fairly humdrum entities, not notably
miraculous at all, that transcend Turing machinehood. An analog computer,
for instance, isn't a Turing machine.[14] In his book, Penrose remarks that a
human being could well be mentally equivalent to a 'device', just not to a
machine in the particular technical sense of a Turing machine. At first
glance it may not be any more inspiring to be a device than a machine—to
me, being a device sounds less enticing, because I associate the term with
shoehorns and dental implements—but it is true that devices in Penrose's
sense can answer certain questions that Turing machines can't. What is
unknown is whether we humans can answer these questions.

Scientists differ on this point, but several things are clear. Penrose has
shown that you are forced into contradictions if you assume the following
three things: that you are equivalent, in your mathematical skills, to some
Turing machine; that you can know your own program (the list of instructions in your Turing-machine counterpart); and that you can know that your
program is valid, in the sense that it never delivers the wrong answer to any
question. So at least one of these three premises must be rejected—that
much is uncontroversial, and as Penrose says, this result was known to
Turing. But which premise is false? Different master detectives have gathered
these suspects together into one room and unfortunately fingered different
ones as the culprit. For Penrose, the most plausible solution is to deny that
we are machines. Turing instead rejected the idea that our program is strictly
valid. That seems reasonable to me, and if I may offer another opinion of
my own, like Inspector Clouseau barging in to assist Holmes and Poirot,
I would also doubt the premise that we can know our own program in perfect detail. Complete, personal self-knowledge may be impossible even in
principle, whether we are computational machines or supercomputational
devices, because it would lead to self-referential paradoxes (but this limit to
self-knowledge poses no problem for computational neuroscience: there is
usually no self-referential danger in my running a complete simulation of
someone else, or of a 'typical human').

So no one has yet managed to demonstrate any logical inconsistency in the idea of exact computational simulations or replicas of human brains, though of course no one has proved its consistency either. Personally, I would take my chances on a computational brain transplant if my own equipment were about to fail. I picture this happening in a futuristic world that has seen major advances in robotics and sensorimotor theory: a competent-looking, well-funded team of scientists tells me, 'Dr Tweed, based on your quantum brain scans, your breathalyzer test, and the questionnaire you filled out, we've constructed an electronic copy of your brain that matches all its input–output performance; it behaves just like you in any situation, or at least it is the best computational approximation to you. So if your brain is in fact a machine—we're still not quite sure about that—the copy will be perfect. But if your brain isn't a machine, there'll be something missing from the copy, because it's merely a computational approximation to you.' I would accept their offer.

Penrose, lying in the next hospital bed, would presumably feel that life as a purely computational being is no worthwhile life at all. He would fear the loss of his supercomputational math skills. He might also wince at the thought of an automaton walking around introducing itself as Penrose at gatherings and making innumerable gaffes owing to its limited, computational nature.

Would I, in my computational form, be missing important marbles? If I noticed some failing—if I walked around stiff-limbed like a wind-up toy, or if, when anyone made a joke, I stared at them and said 'Does not compute' in a buzzy voice—I would pay a lot of money for an upgrade to a supercomputational version of myself. But we can be sure that nothing that grotesque would happen. It is a mathematical theorem that, even if my brain were supercomputational, still its sensorimotor performance over any finite stretch of my life could be mimicked to arbitrary precision by a computational replica. It is equally uncontroversial that a replica could approximate, as closely as you like, what I would do in an arbitrarily large and varied range of hypothetical or future situations, including ones that resemble, arbitrarily closely, anything I could ever experience over any finite span of time. The replica would show by its behavior whatever insight and creativity and morality I would, so even these sorts of traits are within reach of a computational being. So computational replicas might misrepresent the underlying processes in a non-computational brain, but they might also provide useful insights. In this regard, the situation in neuroscience is no different from that in physics, where every successful theory so far has been amenable to simulation on computers, but where any one of these theories might be merely a numerically close approximation to a reality whose essence is quite different and non-computational. That risk is always with us, but there is little reason to think that it is any more troublesome for brain theory than for any other branch of science.

The inscrutability of networks

It is simply beyond us to understand the brain without help from computers. This point has become clear thanks to work on simulated neural networks. These networks, modeled loosely on the known structure of the brain, are webs of little operators called neurons which influence one another via connections called synapses. Setting aside for the moment the 100 billion cells of the human brain, suppose you are dealing with a network of just ten neurons, and suppose that each neuron is fully described by just a few parameters, say the strengths of a few synapses. Suppose further that the network has learned to do multiplication; it takes two inputs and yields as output their product. I apologize if this isn't a very interesting thing for a network to do, but for the sake of clarity it is useful to start simple, and leave for later the construction of a network that predicts the stock market.

Presented with a complete wiring diagram of the trained network, you would have no hope of discerning what the network does. Unless you programmed the data into a computer simulation, or did the equivalent and lengthy computation with pencil and paper, you wouldn't see that the network is a multiplier.

Things would be worse if you didn't have the network specifications handed to you, but had to deduce them by observing the individual neurons while the network was in operation. Suppose you are dealing with a network of so-called sigmoid neurons, which roughly mimic the behavior of real nerve cells. Each simulated neuron receives a number of inputs, weights them—that is, multiplies each input by some factor—and adds them together. The neuron's firing rate is a nonlinear, saturating function of the sum; that is, a graph of firing rate versus the sum of the weighted inputs isn't a straight line but a curve that flattens out at both ends. Over the middle range, firing rate rises as the sum increases, but above and below the middle range it saturates, never straying outside certain upper and lower bounds—no firing rates above 1000 spikes per second, say, or below zero. Given a multiplier network made of ten of these neurons, you could record the activities of all the cells, but in none of them would you ever see a multiplicative interaction, a case where two inputs to a single neuron were multiplied together by that neuron. The multiplicative processing is a property of the network as a whole, not of the individual cells, all of which simply add together their weighted inputs and apply a nonlinearity.

Real neurons are more complex than these sigmoid cells—there is some justice in the argument that the simulations should be called 'Nooral Networks', by analogy with 'Froot Loops'—but that doesn't alter the point. Whatever the properties of the cells, the computation performed by the network as a whole usually won't resemble the computations performed by its individual units. Any one neuron is a minuscule cog in the works of a vast machine. We can't expect to see network properties in the behavior of single cells. At best we may be able to deduce the network's function by combining data from many cells.

Polling neurons

It takes a lot of single-cell data to reveal the overall function of a network. Cell recording isn't like polling before an election. Pollsters can obtain accurate predictions by sampling relatively tiny numbers of voters and asking each of them just a few questions, but this works only because the amount of information being sought is tiny. Information is measured in bits, where one bit is the amount you get from a correct answer to one yes-or-no question involving equally likely alternatives (more generally, it is the *most* information you can reliably obtain with a yes-or-no question—see Chapter 10). So if there are four candidates in an election, and you want to predict the winner, you are seeking at most two bits of information, because you could single out one candidate with just two yes-or-no questions. Your first question could be 'Will either Candidate I or II win?'. Depending on the answer, your second question might be 'Will II win?' or 'Will IV win?', and whatever the answer, it will single out one victor. Of course you can't simply ask these two questions, because prior to election day no one will be able to answer them with certainty; so you may question many people, but still the information you are forecasting is at most two bits.

If you are polling for some numerical datum, such as the average height of men in the European Union, say to the nearest centimeter, still you are seeking only a tiny quantity of information. Even before you knock on your first door, tape-measure in hand, you can be confident that the average height will lie between about 157 and 188 cm, so at a resolution of 1 cm there are at most 32 possible average heights. As in a short game of Twenty Questions, you can distinguish among 32 possibilities using at most five yes-or-no questions, which means that the information you seek amounts to no more than five bits. By contrast, the amount of single-cell information we need to specify the function of a neural network is enormous.

How enormous is it? How much single-cell data do we need to work out the action of the network as a whole? In the worst case we should expect that, to get even a rough idea of what a network does, we will have to specify the input–output properties of almost every one of its cells. The problem is that almost identical networks, A and B, can have entirely different functions. Returning to the example of ten-cell networks, it is a simple matter to devise two such networks where nine of the ten neurons are identical in all details, all input connections and synaptic strengths, except for their projections on to the one final, output neuron, but where these few differences, confined to the final, output stage, are enough to alter completely the functions of the networks, for instance making one perform multiplication and the other addition. There is no way, by recording from any of the nine cells besides the output one, to tell which network, A or B, we are in. No study of these nine neurons, however complete, can ever tell us whether we are looking at a multiplying or an adding network.

Constructing these networks A and B is a simple matter. Neural networks can be taught, by methods I will discuss later, to approximate almost any mathematical operation. To generate networks A and B, just train a single network C consisting of eleven cells: a set of nine neurons feeding two further output cells, the whole network being driven by two input signals. Train the network so that the activity of one output neuron equals the product of the two inputs while that of the other output neuron is the *sum* of those same inputs. Networks A and B are each obtained simply by omitting one of the output neurons. In the combined network, C, the nine non-output neurons may each be doing two things. Each may contribute to the multiplication of the two inputs and also to the addition. We should be prepared for the possibility of similar, double-duty or multiple-duty neurons in the real brain. In that sense, a single neuron may be a cog in two or more separate machines, contributing to separate tasks as different as multiplication and addition.

I deliberately set out to make networks A and B confusable, but the problem exists, in a less extreme form, even without that sort of contrivance. In most sensorimotor networks, you can alter a small proportion of the connections and obtain a network that does something quite different. You could argue that natural selection has organized the brain in a way that avoids this problem, because it wants the brain to be robust. It doesn't want the loss of a single neuron to alter completely some sensorimotor function. But the problem is hard to escape. If I snip the network's connections from its sensor, or to its muscle, for example, I drastically change its function. One defense is to have a lot of connections—a lot of sensory cells and muscle fibers and a lot of neurons joining them—so that the loss of one element is less devastating. This the brain does, but by multiplying components in this way it doesn't necessarily make life easier for scientists trying to analyze its operation. Given almost any sensorimotor network, then, you can know a great deal about it and still not know what it is doing. Deducing network function from neurons requires a lot of data, and a lot of computer power to piece the data together.

We may not need computers to work out rough, qualitative facts about a network. If we don't care whether the network adds two variables x and y or multiplies them, but only whether it processes x and y as opposed to some other variables, u, v, w, and z, then simple observation may suffice. We may not need computers to discover that the cells in a network are influenced by light or by sound. It may be harder to do the opposite, to rule out an influence, showing for example that certain cells are completely unaffected by light shining in the eyes, because it is always possible that the influence appears only under conditions we haven't thought of testing in our experiments. Influences can be masked by multiplicative interactions; if a neuron's activity equals the product of variables x and y, and if x happens to be zero while you are doing your test, then y will appear to have no effect on the cell because the product xy will always be zero, regardless of what y does. Despite that danger, though, single-cell recording can reveal a lot about the qualitative inputs to networks in the brain. It can also help us understand the operation of individual neurons. But as soon as we take the next step, trying to work out what the whole network is doing with its inputs, we are in a realm of complexity where progress is impossible without computer guidance.

Equivalence

If a single network can do more than one thing, it is also true that many different networks can all do the same thing. Changing the parameters of a network usually changes the operation it performs, but not always, because there are usually equivalent parameter sets, sets that result in exactly the same overall operation. In most simulated networks, and likely in parts of the brain, many different neurons are potentially interchangeable. They may all do different jobs, but they all share a basic plan, so each can learn to do the job of any other, usually by changing its synaptic strengths. So if you have a layered network of this sort of equipotential cell, you can switch any two neurons in any one layer without changing the operation of the network at all: let neuron A have all the input connections and output connections of neuron B and vice versa. And apart from this sort of precise equivalence, there is a huge gray area of different network arrangements that perform approximately the same task. If you train the same network repeatedly to do the same job, starting from different random sets of synaptic weights, you usually arrive at different final networks, but their performance is often nearly identical. It is possible that the same thing happens in the brain. When you return to an activity, say tennis, after a long layoff, as your skills improve again, your sensorimotor circuitry may adopt a configuration that differs from the one it had when last you were at the top of your game. So there is no one-to-one correspondence between microscopic configurations and network performance. Instead there is an abstract correspondence that is likely incalculable without computer support.

Exploiting order

A network may contain regularities that simplify its analysis. Primary visual cortex, for instance, is widely believed to consist of 'pinwheels'.[15, 16] Each pinwheel consists of a large number of cells, all of which respond to illumination over about the same patch of retina. Each cell is an orientation detector, firing most vigorously when its patch of retina sees lines or edges of light oriented at its preferred angle. Within any one pinwheel are cells that cover the whole gamut of orientations; as we move around the pin-wheel's perimeter we encounter cells responding to a smooth progression of angles. Moving across the cortex we traverse a quilt of pinwheels; in certain monkeys, the entire cortex contains about 15 000 of them, covering the visual field.[16] Obviously this order simplifies the cortex. Once we have recorded enough single-cell data to detect the pinwheel pattern, we may reasonably extrapolate anything we learn about one pinwheel to all the others, saving a lot of time.

Finding and exploiting this sort of regularity will be crucial to analyzing the brain. Historically, though, regularities have been easiest to find and understand nearest the functional peripheries of the brain, nearest the sense organs and the muscles. Further from the periphery, for instance in the visual areas of temporal cortex, the patterns become more obscure. This is just what we should expect, because more elaborate neural processing lies between these areas and the familiar, outside world. Again the lesson is that the further we advance from the periphery, the more we will need computer power to discern the patterns in the brain.

Orthodox math

In the 1960s a man named D. A. Robinson left his old life as an engineer and ran away to become a brain scientist. To his new field he brought a largely new approach, applying to the brain the control theory he had learned as an engineer. He was by no means the only person importing these new techniques, but he was one of the most persuasive and successful in my own subspecialty, which is the control of the eyes, so I grew up in the field hearing of his exploits. At first his ideas were met with skepticism by some of the aboriginal, pre-mathematical inhabitants of the realm he was invading. How naive, some of them felt, to apply engineering analyses to neural questions, as though the brain had been built on an assembly line. But many of Robinson's principles, while they may have been discovered by engineers, apply to all kinds of control systems, including the brain, and they led him to a remarkable series of discoveries, including the neural integrator and the internal feedback loop for rapid eye movements, which I will discuss in later chapters. In the face of these triumphs, his adversaries retreated or switched sides, and now his brand of control-systems modeling is an orthodox part of sensorimotor science. Robinson himself has been named the 'Oculomotor Pope' for his insights into the neural mechanisms that steer the eyes.

But when a defending army's line is broken, it needn't surrender outright. It can fall back and regroup at the next point it considers defensible. Accordingly, some skeptics take Robinson's successes to mean not that mathematics is a useful tool for understanding the brain, but merely that there is some value in Robinson's specific brand of mostly linear control-systems modeling. Other types of mathematics are still rejected as outlandish. Surprisingly, this ban sometimes includes the powerful optimization ideas that were used by an earlier and even greater sensorimotor pioneer, Hermann von Helmholtz. Helmholtz's reputation is enormous, but except in his few popular lectures he didn't worry about making himself comprehensible to a wide readership. To neuroscientists unfamiliar with mathematics he showed no mercy, expounding his message in dense blocks of equations, and so they have respectfully ignored him.

Where does a math-skeptical neuroscientist draw the line between acceptable and unacceptable mathematics? Often the criterion seems to be a feeling about the 'naturalness' of a mathematical concept. Familiar concepts such as numbers are deemed natural, so a proposal that fibers in the brain convey numerical information is considered sensible. Vectors (see the Glossary) also are acceptable, probably because it is recognized that they can be represented by sets of numbers. Less familiar mathematical objects like quaternions and tensors have been shunned as unbiological, though in fact they are equally easy to represent in networks. On this view, numbers and vectors are the cotton and wool of the mathematical world, as against the polyester and spandex of quaternions and tensors. But this prejudice has no mathematical foundation. Its exponents are simply mistaking familiarity for naturalness. Mathematical concepts that are well established or remembered from schooldays are natural, the rest are offensive to Mother Nature. On closer acquaintance, though, the new concepts are as natural as the older ones. And so-called natural concepts are often the product of years of ingenious labor by human mathematicians. The modern definition of a vector, for instance, took shape over a couple of centuries. Even the intuitively clear notion of velocity was a long time in the making. That concept is a good one for illustrative purposes because we will need it later, when we discuss dynamics and degrees of freedom.

The invention of velocity

To find your average velocity over the last hour, you draw a vector from your location an hour ago to your current location, and divide that vector by the elapsed time, 1 hour. One hour ago I was likely sitting in this same chair, so my average velocity has been zero kilometers per hour (I have been pacing and getting up for snacks, so my average *speed*—the path length of my strolling divided by an hour—is not zero, but that is another concept). In general, average velocity over any time interval is displacement divided by time.

That is average velocity, but what is *instantaneous* velocity? Intuitively, most of us feel that an arrow or a rocket has some velocity at every moment, and at least since Isaac Newton, the concept of instantaneous velocity has played a central role in physics. Newton was vague in his definition of instantaneous velocity, treating it as the ratio of an infinitesimal displacement to an infinitesimal time interval. But infinitesimal numbers—defined as quantities smaller than any positive real number but larger than zero—were for centuries believed by most people to be logically impossible. So it seemed that instantaneous velocity would have to be defined as displacement over a zero time interval, or in other words, how far you traveled in no time, divided by that time. But that calculation made no sense, as zero divided by zero is mathematically indefinite. Throughout the 18th century, mathematicians and physicists made daily use of the concept of instantaneous velocity, despite having no sensible definition for it. The philosopher Bishop Berkeley, who was fed up with scientists' smart remarks about the irrationality of religion, seized upon this embarrassment in his 1734 book *The Analyst,* an exposé of the logical holes at the core of science. This particular hole wasn't repaired until 1829, when Augustin Cauchy used his new concept of a limit to devise a rigorous definition of instantaneous velocity. Cauchy's definition is now taught to students in calculus courses the world over, but it is still probably the most logically complex notion that the students have come across to that point, and at first it doesn't seem particularly natural. In the 1960s, the mathematician Abraham Robinson,[17] no relation, I think, to the Oculomotor Pope, managed to devise a consistent concept of infinitesimal numbers with which he forged a definition of velocity closer in spirit to Newton's ideas. So now we have more than one logically impeccable, functionally equivalent definition of instantaneous velocity. But finding them took a lot of effort by Cauchy, Abraham Robinson, and a long line of other analysts. To call velocity a 'natural' concept is to ignore that work. Equally misguided, and more harmful, is to reject tensors and quaternions and so on as artificial inventions and therefore unbiological. There is no useful distinction here between organic and synthetic math. Everything in mathematics is a hard-won piece of human culture that may be useful if it mirrors some aspect of the world.

Nonlinear thinking

The concept that neuroscientists most misguidedly cherish as natural is linearity. In a way this is odd, because in popular culture the word linear is often a term of disparagement: 'linear' thinking is rigid and blinkered. But in mathematics, an operation is said to be linear if it preserves sums and scaling. If you double the input, for instance, the output doubles. An example of a linear operation is multiplication by any constant, say by 5: an input of 2 yields output 10; doubling the input to 4 doubles the output to 20. Why the name, *linear*? If a variable, y, is a linear function of x, then a graph of y versus x will be a straight line through the origin—that is, through the cross-hair of the graph where both x and y equal 0. So the name is slightly misleading: a straight-line graph that doesn't pass through the origin is not a linear function in the mathematical sense.

Strictly linear operators are rare in nature, but when they do show up they are welcome, because they can be represented using easy mathematics. D. A. Robinson made heavy use of mathematical tools called Laplace transforms, which are wonderfully efficient for describing processes that unfold in time, but they apply only when the unfolding obeys certain linear rules. Unfortunately, few operators in the brain are linear, because the brain is a network of nonlinear neurons. Actually, our nonlinearity is fortunate for us, because we would never have survived with linear brains. As I will explain in Chapter 5, only nonlinear neurons allow universal approximation. They can connect themselves up to perform a close approximation to a linear operation when it is useful to do so, but they have no preference for linear operations, and they can perform an enormous range of nonlinear operations besides. So our nonlinearity allows us to approximate whatever brain operations are optimal for a given task. But it does make things mathematically inconvenient for people studying the brain. Some scientists are reluctant to give up familiar, linear techniques merely because they don't apply. Some cling to linear models of neural systems even when optimization arguments show that the system couldn't begin to function correctly if it were linear, and when the experimental data point to an optimized, nonlinear design. Of course I am not saying that linearity should be avoided, merely that it shouldn't be pursued for its own sake. Where optimization arguments reveal an advantage to linearity, I would expect to find roughly linear processing in the brain.

We can't expect the brain to accommodate itself to our mathematics. We have to choose our mathematics to mirror the brain, as Helmholtz did when he applied optimization theory to sensorimotor questions. More generally, we can't rely on neuronal mechanisms fitting any of our preconceived ideas, because our intuitions about the microscopic activity in the brain can't be trusted. As we evolved in the African Rift Valley, we had little call to analyze the internal workings of vast neural networks, so we never evolved instincts for doing so, unless you count our general instinct for analytical thought. We had to interact with other network-controlled entities—with other humans and animals—so we did develop a keen intuition for sensorimotor behavior, but not for the microscopic mechanisms behind that behavior. In matters of implementation, we can't expect our preconceptions to carry us very far. We will have to be flexible, and let the logic of the subject matter drive our choice of new concepts, even if it drives us into strange new realms of mathematics.

Chapter 4

Genome for a network

Even if there is no objection in principle to the idea of simulating a mind inside a computer there are still practical problems, the main one being the sheer complexity of the brain. It helps that we will be starting with simpler neural systems and leaving the details to computers, but what matters most is that we find patterns in the brain's organization to simplify our descriptions. Our role models might be the image-compression algorithms like JPEG, which exploit regularities in pictures to shrink graphics files. Grander examples are the laws of physics, which are regularities that simplify our description of the universe. But some people doubt that many such simplifying principles exist for the brain. The law-based approach that has worked so well in physics may not work in neuroscience, they say, because the brain may be its own simplest description. It may be incompressible, like a computer file that has already been zipped once and can't be zipped any further. In this chapter I will suggest that we can learn from the example of natural selection, which has managed to zip the brain dramatically, into a self-extracting file in the form of an egg cell, though I will also urge that the egg cell's lessons have to be interpreted with care.

The first thing to notice is that complexity depends on viewpoint. Roughly speaking, the complexity of a thing is the length of the shortest recipe for making it. So the complexity of any one thing varies tremendously depending on the ingredients we have to work with and on the basic operations we take as single steps in our recipes. It is a simple job, for example, to construct a supercomputer if the pieces we have to work with are bolts, a screwdriver, the computer's casing, and the rest of the computer without its casing.

In geometry, the ultimate building blocks are usually taken to be points. On this view, shapes like circles are complex objects, made of an infinity of points arranged according to certain rules. But it is possible to do as the mathematician Alfred North Whitehead did, and redevelop geometry from a different viewpoint, taking circles as the building blocks. Points are then defined as limits of infinite sequences of nested circles, where all the circles sit inside all the preceding ones like matryoshka dolls. In this scheme, it is the circles that are simple and the points that are complex.

In computer animation, figures and landscapes and other forms are typically constructed by gluing together many small triangles or other flat polygons. In this scheme, a sphere is approximated by a multifaceted polyhedron, like a cut diamond. To get a smoother surface, we need more facets. So a perfect sphere is a complex object, made of infinitely many polygons. But it is possible to take spheres as our basic objects, in which case cubes and pyramids and other polyhedra are complex. Our assignments of complexity depend on what we see as our basic ingredients and the basic operations we perform on them.

In complexity theory, the usual basic operations are those of Turing machines. As we have seen, these are idealized computers that can handle data streams—strings of zeros and ones—of unbounded length. They can run simple programs containing just a few instructions, or programs of immense complexity. As a definition, we say that a string is simple if it can be computed by a Turing machine running a small program, and complex if it can be computed only with large programs. This measure of complexity is called algorithmic information content.[18, 19] It applies, strictly speaking, only to Turing machines and strings of zeros and ones. To apply the idea to the brain, we need to adapt it.

The unzipped brain

Because we want to simulate the brain in a computer, we will take as our basic operations the usual ones that are built into computer programming languages, for instance arithmetic operations, logic, and loops. So our basic operations are essentially the same as those in the strict definition of algorithmic information content, but we will replace the strings of zeros and ones by objects more like brains, namely neural networks. The network's complexity will be the length of the shortest program that generates it.

As a first stab at quantifying the brain's complexity, I will simply count up its elements. Obviously this is a naive approach because it ignores any patterns in the network that might allow a briefer description, but it conveys the magnitude of the challenge, and the importance of finding such patterns.

Even in my naive calculation I will allow myself some simplifications, so as to make the task more clearly definable. As I am concerned with programming a brain, not with powering it, cooling it, oiling it and so on, I will ignore those features of neurons that are shared by most other cells in the body, such as the metabolic machinery of power supply, waste removal, and so on. I will assume further that all functionally important differences between neurons are in their synapses, so that I can specify a network merely by specifying the synaptic connections; this assumption is true for most artificial neural networks, and probably false for the real brain, where other neuronal properties, such as membrane dynamics remote from the synapses, likely make a functional difference. But even with these simplifications, the pre-zipping complexity of the brain will be daunting enough.

A human brain contains about 100 billion neurons.[20] If an average neuron receives 3000 synapses, then we have 300 trillion, or 3×10^{14}, synapses in all. How complex is each synapse? How many variants are possible, with different neurotransmitters and receptors, different numbers of release vesicles and receptor sites, that might make a discernible difference to brain function? It is hard to say, but we are surely safe in assuming that there are at least 1000 possible kinds of synapse in the brain. If there are 1000 kinds of synapse, then it can take up to 10 bits of information to specify a synapse completely (2 to the 10th power is 1024, so we can distinguish among 1024 possibilities with 10 yes-or-no questions). If we need 10 bits of information to describe each synapse then we need 3×10^{15} bits to describe all the synapses in the brain. If instead there are a million different possible kinds of synapse, then we need 20 bits to specify each one, and the total bit count doubles, to 6×10^{15}.

But these bits are far from a full description of the brain, because they don't tell us which neurons the synapses are connecting. Obviously this is critical because different patterns of connection will yield networks with entirely different behaviors. So what we really want is a wiring diagram of the brain. This can be described using an array of 100 billion rows (one for each neuron) and the same number of columns. The entry in the ith row and jth column of the array describes the synapse from the ith to the jth neuron (if there is no synapse between them, place a zero in the array; we ignore the complication that several synapses may connect any two neurons). Assuming, again, 10 bits per synapse, the total number of bits in our description comes to 100 billion squared times 10, or 10^{23}.

We can save bits by exploiting the fact that the array of synapses is sparse: most of its entries are zeros, because most cells in the brain don't talk to each other directly. There are techniques for compressing the information in sparse arrays. Using the best compression techniques available, we can reduce the description to about 1.7×10^{16} bits. That much information would fit on about 20 000 hard drives of 100 gigabytes each. If memory devices continue to advance at their current rates, then by the time you read this it may be possible to store a brain in this form on a pen drive, but all the same, the volume of data is staggering, and the motivation is strong to discover a simplifying description.

The genome

We know that natural selection has discovered a way to create brains from remarkably little, essentially a small amount of genetic material enclosed in a single egg cell. Can we compute how far natural selection has managed to zip the brain?

Inside the egg, deoxyribonucleic acid, or DNA, holds the instructions for building the brain. DNA carries its message in a sequence of base pairs. Given that the order of the two bases in the pair carries information, there are four kinds of pair—adenine-thymine, thymine-adenine, cytosine-guanine, guanine-cytosine—so in effect the DNA message is written in an alphabet of four letters. Four different letters can be distinguished with two yes-or-no questions, so each base pair carries up to two bits of information.[21] Our entire genome, including the small bits in the mitochondria, contains about three billion base pairs, which provide an information capacity of six billion bits in human DNA as a whole. According to molecular biologists only about five per cent of this information seems to be used.[22] In that case the biologically relevant information content of human DNA falls to something like 300 million bits. Rounding up liberally, we can say that the genetic instructions for building a human being amount to some 50 megabytes, which is probably fewer than Microsoft used to code the talking paperclip in Word. So the genetic specifications for a human brain are likely no more complex than this.

Stray bits

Some bits of information are missing from this account. For one thing, in the cells of a human body, base pairs in the DNA may be linked to other small molecules, for instance methyl groups, in which case the information is being carried by an alphabet of more than four letters. Besides the four base pairs, there are many variants of these four, labeled with methyl groups or other tags, like accidentals attached to letters in an alphabet. If DNA works with an alphabet of more than four letters, then our estimate of its information content will have to be raised. It seems that the tags are used mainly to inactivate harmful genes and to turn genes on and off in particular tissues, so that liver genes are on in the liver and off in the kidney. Most of them, it is believed, are cleared or reset in the eggs and sperm, so they don't convey much hereditary information to the next generation. But if it turns out that many such labels do persist in germ cell DNA, then our estimate of its information content may have to be raised.

Another issue is that the genome might conceivably include other cellular materials besides DNA. The defining feature of genetic material is that changes there can be passed on to later generations. Evolution is driven by small changes, because large changes are usually catastrophic. But the only small changes that pass to future generations are those in the genome. A small change in the DNA of an egg or sperm cell is passed on to its descendants, but a similar small change in a membrane lipid, cytoplasmic protein, or sugar will not usually be passed on. That lipid, protein, or sugar molecule will eventually decay and will be replaced by the cellular machinery which is directed by the instructions in the DNA. This is what it means to say that DNA is the medium of heredity, which is a central dogma of modern biology. But of course the dogma may be mistaken, and probably it is slightly oversimplified. Freeman Dyson and others argue that metabolic systems could carry hereditary information.[23-25] It has been suggested that prions—the protein molecules that cause encephalopathies like scrapie, kuru, and mad-cow disease—may do the same. And it is widely accepted that chemicals other than DNA served as genetic material in our evolutionary past, before DNA took over.[23-26] Future research may reveal other present-day carriers of hereditary information, in which case the complexity of the genome will have to be recalculated, but the current consensus seems to be that any such revisions will be minor, because the principal carrier is DNA. And in that case the genetic instruction list for building the brain may stay on the order of 50 megabytes.

Did selection zip the brain?

Does it serve a purpose to make the genome so compact? The point is probably not to save space in the cell nucleus. DNA doesn't weigh much or take up much room, so there is probably little reason to compress the genome on that account. And extra DNA may even serve some function, promoting chemical reactions or maybe shielding the rest of the DNA from radiation. Amebas, lilies, and salamanders have far more DNA than humans do, so presumably they are carrying around more genome that they really need, again suggesting that natural selection isn't trying to reduce DNA content.

But even if natural selection doesn't care about the total amount of DNA in the cell, it may still try to minimize the length of the coding sequence: the stretches of DNA that are translated into proteins, or in other words that contain genes. Every time a cell divides, its DNA must be copied. The longer the coding sequence, the more likely it is that an error will be made in copying it. When it exceeds a certain length, copying errors are almost guaranteed, and then natural selection becomes ineffective because particularly adaptive DNA sequences aren't passed on to offspring but are ruined through copying errors. How long the coding sequence can grow before this happens depends on the fidelity of the copying process. It may be that the length of our coding sequence is near some optimum set by our copying fidelity,[25] and that this is the motivation for compressing the genome.

There are two broad principles the genome might use to compress information about the brain. One is to exploit regularities in the brain, in much the same way that a graphics compression algorithm exploits regularities in an image. If a large number of neurons are largely alike, the genome might code just one blueprint for them all. If every pinwheel in the primary visual cortex has to be wired in much the same way, code just one pinwheel. Other examples may involve subtler regularities. Fractals like the Mandelbrot set aren't obviously redundant, yet they can be generated by very simple programs. Similarly abstract order may also exist in the brain.

The other principle is to build a protobrain that can draw information from the environment, or in other words learn. We know that much of the information in the brain does come from the environment rather than from the genes alone. For one thing, the genetic specifications of course exclude all the memories in the mature brain, all knowledge acquired after conception. This point is sometimes ignored in movies. In the film *Multiplicity*, an overworked man arranges to be cloned so that he can delegate jobs to himself. Each clone comes to life full-grown, knowing the man's address, the name of his wife, and a lot of other information that wouldn't really be present in his genes. It is true that there are stories about identical twins, reared apart from birth, who share quirks or biographical details—they dress similarly, or they both marry fat lawyers. Still, detailed knowledge of your life isn't specified genetically, but is written into your brain by your experiences. It will never be possible, by DNA testing, to learn in advance the name of the person you will marry. And even apart from personal knowledge of this sort, it is clear that some basic capabilities such as language and vision don't develop properly unless the brain encounters appropriate stimuli at appropriate times.

So genes don't describe a complete brain but rather a protobrain, an entity that, driven by sensory information from the environment, organizes itself into a brain. Probably this is the main lesson to draw from the genome story: that in our quest for simplifying order we should focus on how the brain builds itself based on inputs from its environment. But can we squeeze any quantitative encouragement out of this story? We have seen that the genome holds the instructions for a protobrain in just 50 megabytes. Can we take this to mean that a program of just 50 megabytes might be able to drive the development of a brain in a computer? Unfortunately there are problems with this idea.

Information in the egg

The problems begin with the fact that information content can be measured only within a context of possibilities. Knowing that 50 megabytes of DNA suffice to specify a protobrain doesn't mean that 50 megabytes of computer code will do the same, because the range of possibilities—the set of things that could be built, given the right instructions—may be quite different for DNA in a fertilized egg cell than for code in a personal computer. If the DNA instructions are being read by a machine that has been specially designed to build viable brains, then it might need far fewer bits than would a machine with no bias toward building viable brains, such as, presumably, a PC.

Imagine that you are in business with a clockmaker who constructs, by hand, wonderfully intricate chronometers. The clockmaker builds two models of clock, called Model 0 and Model 1. Your job is to travel the world collecting orders for these clocks. Whenever you get an order, you send the information back to your partner. Because you love brevity, your message always consists of just one symbol, either a 0 if the order is for a Model 0 or a 1 for a Model 1. A truly naive observer might conclude that the clocks being ordered are very simple, because they can be specified by a single bit of information, a 0 versus a 1. But by any sensible measure, the clocks are in fact highly complex. The extra information comes from the clockmaker, who over years of practice has learned to build his intricate machines, and who has devised with you the simple 0-1 code. It is possible that a similar situation holds in human embryology. A simple DNA message of just 50 megabytes may suffice to specify a protobrain only because its message is read by the immensely complex egg cell, which is a specialized brain-building machine (the contribution of the wider world outside the egg seems relatively small: a bird's egg builds a bird without apparently requiring much from its surroundings, until the chick hatches, beyond a certain temperature and atmosphere). The moral is that we may need a far more complex message to get a PC to construct a brain, given that a PC isn't specialized for brain building.

Of course there is an important difference between the clockmaker reading your messages and the egg cell reading its genome. The genome contains the instructions for building an entire body, including the eggs themselves, whereas your messages do not contain the instructions for building clockmakers. The moral of the story would have been different if you had sent not single 0's or 1's but zipped, self-extracting clockmaker programs, and your messages were received not by a wise old craftsman but by a robot—a general-purpose robot who had been designed with no thought of clockmaking in particular. In that case it would have been reasonable to say that the complexity of your messages reflected the complexity of the resulting clocks. Can we use considerations like these to resurrect the idea that the complexity of a protobrain on a PC might amount to just 50 megabytes?

It is true that the genome contains instructions for building eggs. Not in the sense that a naked DNA molecule lying on a sidewalk could absorb atoms from the air and construct an egg cell around itself, but in the sense that every adaptation in the egg cell is ultimately due to an adaptation in the DNA. This is the crucial point. Consider the DNA–egg cell complex and imagine its evolution through the ages. Wind back the clock far enough and we arrive, we think, at a simple DNA molecule inside a protein casing or lipid bubble. Since then, almost every favorable change, almost every adaptation that has made the system better at building brains has been a change in the DNA sequence.

If we imagine a primordial DNA string, randomly arranged, then every adaptation consists of a change, addition, or deletion of a base pair. At most three billion such changes are needed to get from a random distribution to the one we have today, at most three billion decisions by natural selection. Can we say that each decision adds two bits of information, and therefore that natural selection injects at most six billion bits of information to transform the random DNA string in its protocell into the modern, functioning DNA–egg complex? We can't, because the order and context of these decisions may also matter. And if order matters, then natural selection had far more than 2-to-the-6-billion possible courses of action, and may therefore have injected far more than 6 billion bits of information. In short, I see no likely prospects for obtaining a quantitative estimate of the complexity of the brain along these lines.

Advantages over the egg

In some ways we can reasonably hope that a brain-building program in a computer may be simpler than the chemical program in a real, embryonic brain. In the computer, a brain can be specified by an array of synapses; as arrays are simple data structures, programming languages must be about as well suited for specifying brains as anything can be. In contrast, think of the complexity of building a brain using chemistry. Think of the riga-marole the developing brain has to go through to guide baby neurons to their correct stations in the brain and to hook them up. From germinal zones around the ventricles, spokes of radial glia stream out, forming, evidently, a sort of framework for neural migration. Then the neurons start marching. In cortical development, the first marchers are the first to stop, forming the deepest layer of cortex. Later arrivals pass through the sheets of earlier pioneers to form more superficial layers. Only after the immature, round neurons reach their appointed places do they send out cytoplasmic feelers, inchoate axons and dendrites, seeking contact with distant cells. In the PC, cells can be placed and connected with a few keystrokes, simply by entering a number into the array that represents the wiring diagram. This shows that brain development is more straightforward in a PC, not necessarily that it can be guided by a simpler program, and presumably the job of specifying a *viable* brain on a PC, as opposed to just any brain, will require complex programming, but it does seem that much of the complication of embryonic development may be avoidable in a PC. And many of the discoveries that natural selection had to program into the egg are known to us already, so they provide pre-existing structure and context for our brain program: metabolism and cell division; the very idea of an adaptive, computational network; sensors for light, sound, motion, and so on; and a muscle-powered skeleton. These observations suggest that a program considerably simpler than an egg cell may be able to specify protobrains in a computer.

Decoding the brain

Even if its complexity is hard to estimate, an egg cell is clearly more compact than the body that unfolds from it, and embryology is a remarkable example of unzipping. What can we learn from this example? Should we take it as our job to decipher the genomic code, or in other words to try to simulate the molecular processes by which DNA directs the construction of the brain? At the moment I see this as a wonderful project for somebody else. For myself, I hope there is an easier road to understanding the brain. One crucial point is that the genome is a program whose basic operations are chemical reactions about which we know very little; what we want is a program based on the familiar logical operations of digital computers. Another problem with decoding the genome is that the genes act through a phenomenally complex web of chemical reactions whose details are almost unknown. Does this contradict my claim that the genome is a remarkably simple encoding of the brain? No, because there is more than one meaning to the word simple.

Run-time complexity

Returning to the example of Turing machines computing strings of ones and zeros, I said that a string is simple if it can be computed by a small program. A string of this type is said to have a small algorithmic information content. But a string that is simple in this sense may in another sense be complicated to realize. The tiny program that generates it may take a long time to run through its calculation, billions or trillions of steps. In a PC, a one-line program can drive a computer round and round a loop a billion times, or for ever. Considerations like these have led to different measures of complexity, such as logical depth, which is, roughly, the time it takes to compute a string using the smallest program that does so.[27-29] For instance, fractals like the famous Mandelbrot set, with their infinitely nested structure, appear highly complex, but their algorithmic information content is actually very small because the program you need to draw one of these shapes takes only a few lines of code on a computer. The number of computational steps may be large, though, if you want to draw the set at high resolution, so the picture is logically deep. That one and the same object can be simple in one sense and complex in another isn't a flaw in our analysis of the concept of complexity. Rather it is an interesting discovery that the vague, everyday notion of complexity, when it is made precise, splits into a number of distinct technical concepts, including algorithmic information content and logical depth.

Now the run-time complexity of the chemical processes that turn genetic instructions into a brain is enormous. Simulating how even one protein molecule will fold up on itself is a job for a supercomputer. IBM is building a new machine just for this purpose, called Blue Gene, that will make its previous showpiece, Deep Blue, look like a chess-playing cash register. So it is out of the question, now and maybe for ever, to try to simulate brain development at the atomic level, which is what we would have to do if we wanted to simulate a mutation in our DNA and predict its consequences for the brain, or if we wanted to test new drugs by simulation.

Instead of simulating brain development atom by atom we could do it gene by gene, or molecule by molecule. If 40 000 genes contribute to building the brain, we could define 40 000 variables, one for each gene, and a few times that many further variables for gene products and other molecules that aren't gene products but are ingested or arise through chemical reactions. Given a huge archive of experimental data describing the rates and products of the reactions between all these molecules we might be able to simulate development. Obviously a whole-brain simulation of this sort is a long way off, but so it is on any approach. More restricted simulations of the role of one or a few genes in brain development may be practical in the near future.

Another approach would be to forget about mechanisms altogether, and just look for correlations between genes and brains. We leap over the complex chemistry of neural development and simply correlate genomes with finished brains. In this way, molecular biologists have identified the genes for many diseases without yet understanding much about how the genes cause their damage. Decoding the genome in this way is like coming across a machine with a control console of 40 000 knobs and switches, none of them labeled, and trying to work out what each one does. Some switches will have a clearly discernible job, turning on or off a motor or blinking lamp—these correspond to the easily interpretable genes, in most cases ones that cause massive breakdowns like Huntington disease or cystic fibrosis. But many switches will have subtle, widespread effects on the machine's function that are hard to sort out. From what we know about genetics, it is clear that many switches will appear to have no effect at all, until we discover that turning them on when some other switch is on, and the temperature is within some range, and so on, shuts the machine off entirely, or has other drastic effects. Actually, this machine analogy makes the task seem simpler than it is, because we naturally assume that the machine's control panel was built by humans, and that the knobs and switches correspond to functions that human users find intuitive. But the genome was designed by no one like us, and we can't count on intuition providing much help. I believe there are other ways of looking at the brain where our intuition will be a better guide.

Crypticity and intuition

In some ways the most relevant measure of brain complexity is neither algorithmic information content nor logical depth, but a third measure called crypticity.[27] This, roughly speaking, is logical depth in reverse. Given a string of ones and zeros, crypticity quantifies how long it takes to deduce, from the string, the shortest program that would generate it. In the case of the brain, crypticity measures how much work it will be to deduce a compact description from neural data. I can't begin to estimate the crypticity of the brain, especially as we are interested not in how long an optimally rational being or machine would need to deduce the description given the data but in how long human neuroscientists will need, with all our biases and assumptions and insights.

You can slice a brain conceptually along many different dimensions. In this book I focus on the dimension of performance, so I look at the brain as a set of sensorimotor modules. But you can also slice the brain anatomically, into cortices, tracts, and nuclei, and then study, for instance, the operation of the cerebellum or the thalamus. You can slice the brain chemically, looking at, say, its glutamate or acetylcholine modules. Or you can study the genetic dimension, unraveling what each gene does in the brain. Different dimensions are important for different purposes. For surgery, it may be the anatomical dimension that matters most. For drug and gene therapy, it may be the chemical and genetic dimensions. For rehabilitation, ergonomics, and robotics, the sensorimotor dimension.

But understanding one dimension can shed light on the others. For example, sensorimotor insights can guide us to molecular discoveries. The NMDA receptor is a molecule which, it now seems, may play an important role in learning, but its significance might easily have been missed had not the psychologist Donald Hebb, years earlier, pointed out that a chemical with its properties would be useful for learning.[30] As I will discuss later, it is a safe guess that there are other, intracellular mechanisms critical to learning and brain development that will go unnoticed or unappreciated until theoretical work on self-organizing networks shows us what we should be looking for.

It may be that we can decipher the brain fastest by concentrating first on the easiest dimension, which is performance. We could instead start anatomically, asking for instance what the cerebellum does. But whatever it does, we can't expect that it will be easily expressible in any concepts we have right now because we have had so little experience with enormously complex networks. We are dreaming if we expect to capture in any useful way the role of the cerebellum in a few common-sense terms like 'learning' or 'timing'. As our neuroscience and control theory advance, we will develop more useful concepts, but it may be a long road. Probably the chemical and genetic dimensions will be even harder to comprehend because they involve even more complex and foreign networks of chemical reactions. But when we explore sensorimotor performance, our way is lit by our insight into life as an animal on Earth. We know almost without thinking why our hands have several fingers, why our corneas are clear, why our eyes are rotatable. And, as I will try to show through much of this book, we can with a little thought deduce the reasons for most other sensorimotor facts—why there is a fast neural projection to carry signals from our inner ears to our eyes, why the muscles for our fingers are way up in our forearms, why the biceps inserts near the elbow rather than the wrist, why fast eye movements aren't guided to their targets by vision, why IMAX movies make us feel as though we are moving, and so on.

I suggest, then, that working out the performance dimension of the brain may be a fast way to gather knowledge about the other dimensions. It is as if I were faced with a crossword puzzle where the horizontal words were in English and the vertical words were in Spanish. As my English is good and my Spanish isn't, I would be wise to concentrate on the English words first, even though my aim is to fill in both the rows and the columns. In most crosswords, if I get all the rows I thereby get all the columns, but even if I am dealing with a gappy crossword where the rows don't determine everything in the columns, I would still, as an English speaker, fill in the Spanish words fastest by solving the English ones first. One motivation behind the approach in this book is the idea that the brain is like a gappy, multidimensional crossword puzzle whose easiest dimension is sensorimotor performance.

Chapter 5

The adaptive brain

To cope with an uncertain, changing world, the brain must be able to reprogram itself on the fly. Its sensorimotor systems will do their jobs only if they are correctly tuned, their synapses set to appropriate values. The right setting for each synapse depends on how the other synapses are set, and on the state of the sense organs and the muscles. If a muscle weakens, the neural signals driving it must strengthen to achieve the same motion. But then how does a sensorimotor system stay accurate over a lifetime, as the sensors and muscles, and the body parts moved by the muscles, change with growth, injury, aging, and disease? And how does it tune itself in the first place, in the fetal and infant brain, when the neural circuits encounter the newly formed sensors and muscles for the first time? There is only one way. It manages all this by constantly monitoring and calibrating itself, adjusting its own internal structure to optimize its performance. Working out the mechanisms of biological learning will be one of the most fundamental, unifying achievements in neuroscience. And even before we fully grasp the mechanisms, the mere knowledge that the brain is a self-adjusting system opens a path to understanding it. It suggests that much of the information in the brain may be concentrated in certain master circuits, in the error signals that guide learning. I will argue that networks of bewildering complexity can be made comprehensible if we focus on optimization and error signals.

Simple learning

If you put on prism spectacles that rotate your visual world, say 10 degrees to the right, then your reaching and aiming and trapeze artistry will at first be impaired. If you throw tennis balls at a target, they will hit about 10 degrees too far to the right, where you think the target is. You can apply your reason to the problem, noticing your errors and consciously resolving to aim 10 degrees left. But even if you give the problem no conscious thought, if you just keep hurling balls, your performance will quickly improve as you get used to the new relation between vision and arm control. If you then remove the prism goggles, you will be in trouble again, now throwing 10 degrees too far *left*, and it will take a few minutes before your brain readjusts to life without prisms. In the space of a few minutes, then, your brain recalibrates itself based on a change in its sensory experience.

Thomas Thach and colleagues had people throw while wearing prism goggles.[31] They found that if people practiced overhand throwing they quickly learned to hit the target, but their adaptation didn't usually transfer to underhand throwing. It has been said that this lack of transfer makes sense functionally, because you wouldn't want adjustments to one skill interfering with another. You wouldn't want your golf swing to change when you worked on your tennis serve. But this finding raises some questions about adaptation.

Adaptation depends on the brain running self-diagnostic programs. When a throw goes astray, the problem might be in the eyes, in the arm muscles, or somewhere in between; the diagnostics program should find the problem and correct it or compensate for it. In the prism experiment, the problem is purely visual; a perfect diagnostics package would figure this out and correct it by altering the circuits that localize visual targets in space. This corrected target location would then be used by all motor systems. Ideally, then, underhand throwing (and sidearm throwing, shot-putting, juggling, and so on) would be adapted as soon as overhand throwing was. In this case, where the problem is visual, you would indeed want your golf swing to change with your tennis serve; you would want all your motor systems to act upon the corrected visual information. Thach's results indicate an error in the diagnostics.

Why does the brain make this error? One possibility is that there is no one visual estimate of target location that is used by different motor systems; rather, each motor system has its own estimate. On this view, what happens in Thach's experiment is that the circuits that localize visual targets for the overhand throwing system are repaired, but this does nothing to help underhand throwing. Another idea, more likely I think, is that the brain misdiagnoses the throwing inaccuracy as a problem with arm control rather than vision because, in nature, out-of-practice muscles are more common than prisms covering your eyes.

Given limited information, the brain has to guess at the site of the malfunction. Given a wider range of experience, it should be better able to pinpoint the flaw. If people with prism goggles were allowed to practice a range of visuomotor activities including overhand throwing and pointing and reaching and walking around, but not underhand throwing, their diagnostic routines might eventually deduce that the problem was visual, and adjust underhand throwing even without specific practice.

Ocular maneuvers in the dark

Probably the best-studied example of an adaptive system is the vestibulo-ocular reflex, or VOR. It is also one of the few cases in neuroscience where we can follow a sensorimotor transformation from the sense organs, through the brain, and right back out to the muscles without losing the trail in the neural maze. Your VOR counterrotates your eyes whenever your head turns. Its purpose is to keep your eyeballs as steady as possible relative to your surroundings so that your retinal images don't jiggle when you move. When your head rotates to the right, for instance, your VOR rotates your eyes to the left at the same speed to keep them aimed at their target. So the reflex has much the same job as the steadicam that stabilizes a movie camera or the gyroscope that stabilizes navigational devices on a wave-tossed ship.

But the mechanism is different. A gyroscope reacts mechanically to the motion of the ship, but your eyeballs aren't mechanically rigged to counteract head motion. The eyes of some dolls are rigged to do just that, which is why medical textbooks refer to the VOR as the doll's-eye reflex. (Physicians use it to assess comatose patients—one of the patient's eyes is held open and the head is gently rotated; if the eye doesn't counterrotate like a doll's, then something is wrong in the brainstem.) If you open up a doll's head, you apparently find weights hanging from the backs of the eyeballs, so that gravity can act directly on the eyes. If you open up a human head, you find a different mechanism, where head motion is transduced into neural activity by sense organs and conveyed by the brain to the eye muscles.

Which sense organs are involved? You might guess that they are the eyes themselves, or in other words that the VOR involves visually 'locking on' to an object, keeping your eyes trained on it as your head moves. But that is not how the VOR works—it is not visually driven. We know this because the reflex works in complete darkness, where there is nothing visible to lock on to. To verify this on yourself, try turning your head horizontally, swinging it back and forth through a wide arc. Keep your eyes closed and rest your fingertips lightly on your closed lids. With your fingers you can feel the jittery motion of your eyeballs as they repeatedly turn opposite the head's motion and then reset, flicking back toward their straight-ahead positions. The reason the reflex works in darkness is that it is driven by a sense other than vision.

The sixth sense

Traditional lists and allegorical paintings identify five senses: sight, hearing, touch, taste, and smell. The real list of human senses probably runs to some number between ten and a thousand, depending on how finely you discriminate and on how much conscious awareness you require before you are willing to call a detection system a 'sense'. But those senses beyond the first five didn't make it into the old paintings because they were discovered only later. One of the first additions to the classical list was the sense of self-motion, called the vestibular sense because its organ lies partly within a chamber called the vestibulum in the inner ear. This sense is even starting to gain public recognition. Many people, when asked to name the sixth sense, and when steered away from options like clairvoyance, 'spider sense', and communion with the dead, will eventually say 'balance', and balance is largely a vestibular matter. Besides driving the VOR, the vestibulum provides information to several other reflexes that control our limbs to keep us from falling over. If you stand on one foot with your eyes closed, you can experience these reflexes in action.

Even if we are not normally aware of our vestibular sense, many of us still try to gratify it. Bungee jumps and roller coaster rides are largely vestibular experiences. A roller coaster ride is the vestibular equivalent of music, and designers of these rides are the composers.

But the vestibular sense is one of those things we appreciate best when it is gone. In a 1952 edition of the New England Journal of Medicine there appeared an article called 'Living without a balancing mechanism',[32] written by a physician who lost vestibular function when his inner ear was poisoned by an overdose of the antibiotic streptomycin. Without a VOR, his every movement jarred his vision. He couldn't read signs or recognize friends on the street without stopping and standing still. He couldn't read in bed without bracing himself against the headboard, because his own pulse jiggled his view.

To see for yourself the benefits of having your eyeballs under vestibular and not just visual control, hold your index finger up before your eyes, the palm of your hand toward you. Oscillate your hand back and forth horizontally at a rate of about two cycles per second. You will find that your visual impression of the fast-moving finger is blurred so that your fingerprints aren't clearly visible. But if you hold your finger still and instead oscillate your head at the same rate, you will find your vision much sharper, your fingerprints clear and distinct. Why the difference in perception, given that the relative motion of finger and head is the same in both cases? When the finger moves, you have only visual information about its motion to guide your eye movements (besides your body sense of your own hand motion, which doesn't seem to help much). Visual information normally takes about 100 ms to run from the retina to the visual cortices at the back of the head and then forward, through a series of processing stations, to the motor neurons that move the eyes.[33] This delay is simply too long to let the eye keep up with the oscillating finger. But when your head moves, you have visual and vestibular information about the motion. Vestibular information takes only about one-hundredth of a second to run from the sensors in the inner ear through the brainstem to the muscles that rotate the eyes.[34] Within 10 ms of your head starting to turn rightward, a command for a leftward rotation reaches your eye muscles. Working at this short latency, the VOR has no trouble compensating for the rapid motion of the head.

The labyrinth

This rapid response is driven by an intricate sense organ whose structure reflects the properties of the motion it is designed to detect. In a way, then, knowledge of the laws of motion has been built into our sensors for eons, though these laws were discovered by other parts of our brains only a few centuries ago. For instance, there are two sets of vestibular sensors which detect the two fundamentally different kinds of motion that are available to rigid bodies like the head. The two kinds of motion are called translation and rotation. Translation changes the location of the object, rotation changes its orientation. A train traveling on a straight track, for instance, is changing its location but not its orientation; it is translating but not rotating. A top spinning in place is rotating but not translating. The Earth's yearly motion around the sun is translation, while its circadian turning about its axis is rotation. Translational motion of the head is sensed by the otolith organs, the utricle and saccule, while rotational head motion is sensed by the semicircular canals.

In this chapter I will focus on the canals. These are six fluid-filled tubes, three on each side of the head, each one an almost complete circular hoop. Each canal is filled with a fluid called endolymph and is sealed off at one end by the cupula, a membrane stretched like a drumhead across the lumen of the tube. The three canals on each side of the head lie roughly at right angles to one another, one canal horizontal and the other two in vertical planes. Each canal senses head rotation in its own plane. When the head turns rightward, for instance, the fluid in the horizontal canal on the right side lags the motion, like coffee sloshing backward in a cup in an accelerating car. The fluid presses on the cupula, deforming it. The deformation is sensed by hair cells, whose microscopic hairs, or cilia, extend into the cupular membrane. When pressure deforms the cupula, the hairs bend, altering the voltage across the cell membrane. Nerve fibers contacting the hair cells convey their signals into the brain.

One reason the vestibular sense escaped attention for so long is that its sensors are hidden from view. They are hidden in the labyrinths, which are cavities in the petrous bones of the skull, just medial to the ears. The vestibular organs share this space with the cochlea, the spiral tube that contains the sound-sensitive hair cells that underlie hearing. Why do the vestibular and auditory sensors lie so close together? Because they evolved from the same organ in some remote, aquatic ancestor of ours. Even today, fish have a sort of combined vestibulum–cochlea in the form of the lateral line organ, which consists of tubes open to the surrounding water. Nerve endings detect the flow of water through the tubes, allowing the fish to sense ripples from nearby disturbances, and also its own motion through the water. In humans, their terrestrial cousins, the tubes are filled with endolymph rather than water. They have closed themselves off from the outside world because otherwise we would have endolymph dribbling down our cheeks, which is bad for reproductive success. In humans, the

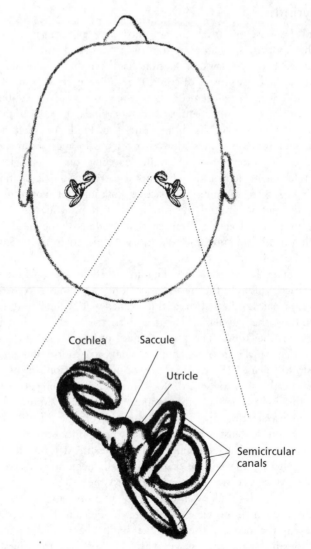

Fig. 5.1 The labyrinth.

twin functions of the lateral line organ are performed by separate sets of tubes: the cochlea detects ripples, also known as sound waves, in the air around us, while the semicircular canals sense our own motion.

The three-neuron arc

What happens in the hundredth of a second between the canals detecting the head motion and the eye muscles contracting to move the eye? Primary vestibular neurons transmit the head-motion signal from the canals into the brainstem. For most natural head motions, the firing rates of these cells reflect the rotational velocity of the head: they carry a head-velocity signal. For instance fibers from the horizontal semicircular canal on the right side of the head fire at a rate proportional to the rightward component of head velocity; fibers from other canals code other components.

Primary neurons synapse with secondary vestibular neurons in the vestibular nucleus in the brainstem. The secondary vestibular neurons in turn project to the motor neurons innervating the eye muscles, influencing them in such a way that the eyes counteract the motion of the head. For example, a secondary vestibular neuron receiving input from the horizontal semicircular canal on the right side of the head—the canal that is excited by rightward head rotation—projects to and activates motor neurons of the lateral rectus muscle of the left eye and the medial rectus muscle of the right eye. Both these muscles rotate the eyes to the left, opposite the head rotation. In this way, the pattern of connections in the brainstem makes eye velocity oppose head velocity. This pathway from canals to muscles through the primary and secondary vestibular neurons and the motor

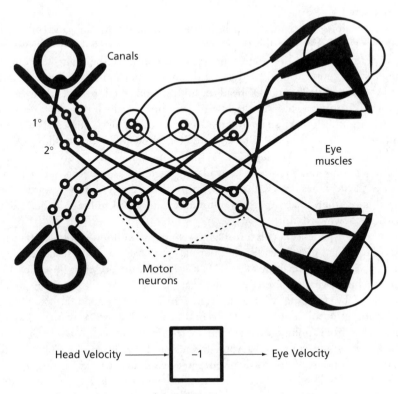

Fig. 5.2 The three-neuron arc of the VOR.

neurons is called the three-neuron arc.[35, 36] But as we will see later, other connections also contribute to the VOR, and vestibular signals are widely distributed in the brain.

Learning in the VOR

Like any sensorimotor system, the VOR will work correctly only if its connections are set to appropriate values, not too strong and not too weak. Otherwise the eyes may turn too fast or too slow, or in the wrong direction, to stabilize vision. The VOR's ability to reprogram itself in the face of malfunctions is impressive.

Vertigo and nystagmus

Floating in the labyrinth, the vestibular sensors are protected from impact, but they can still be damaged, or their connections to the brain severed, by skull fractures, brain tumors, or strokes. If the labyrinth on one side of the head, say the right side, is destroyed, then the normal balance is upset between the vestibular signals from the two sides of the head, and the patient feels a leftward vertigo; that is, an illusory whirling to the left.

One result is nystagmus, which is an alternation of slow and quick eye movements in opposite directions. Because the brain mistakenly believes the head is turning left, it rotates the eyes smoothly to the right to compensate. As the eyes near their rightward limits, they quickly snap back leftwards, towards their straight-ahead positions, and then resume their slower rightward turning. The slow rightward motion is called the slow phase of nystagmus; the quick snap to the left is the quick phase. The name *nystagmus* comes from a Greek word for drowsiness or nodding, as in 'nodding off to sleep'; the idea is that a nodding head shows the same alternating slow–quick pattern as ocular nystagmus, as you can verify in any lecture theater—the drowsy listeners' faces drift slowly down towards their breastbones, then snap up again into momentary wakefulness before resuming their downward drift.

You can experience ocular nystagmus yourself without vestibular damage. For one thing, nystagmus is the normal response to real, sustained head rotation; it was normal nystagmus that you felt under your fingertips during the head-swinging exercise a few paragraphs back. Or you can induce nystagmus by fuddling your vestibular sensors with unnatural stimulation: try whirling in place for twenty seconds, preferably on a soft, grassy surface, away from pointy objects and porcelain figurines. Afterwards, while you lie dizzy on your back, your friends and passers-by can observe the flickering motions of your eyes. You can't see your own nystagmus, even if someone holds a mirror over your face, but you can detect the small lurch of your visual world with every quick phase.

Damaging the right-sided vestibulum, as we have seen, causes nystagmus and leftward vertigo, driven by the unopposed signals from the intact sensors on the left. But over a few days or weeks the nystagmus and vertigo subside. Apparently the centers in the brain that interpret vestibular information become suspicious. They begin to doubt that they have really been whirling to the left for days on end. That motion is inherently implausible, except for performers of acrobatic figure-skating, and it is contradicted by evidence from the other senses; the sense of touch, the sense of limb position, and vision all indicate that the whirling is illusory, that the vestibular signals reporting head rotation are not to be trusted. There follows a period of unconscious introspection or self-diagnosis in which the problem is localized to the relative silence in the right vestibular nucleus. Over time, the cells there increase their firing even with no recovery in the damaged vestibulum; their spontaneous activity builds up until it restores the balance between the right and left sides.[37] The activity may be created by altering the strengths of synapses, as in most simulated learning networks, or by altering other cell properties, such as the ion flux across their membranes, but the end result is that equilibrium is restored. Function doesn't return entirely to normal because the patient is still missing the sensors on one side, but the vertigo and nystagmus disappear, and in many situations the one intact labyrinth can drive an adequate VOR.

Occasionally, the second labyrinth is destroyed after the patient has adapted to the loss of the first. Then the patient relives some of the same story on the second side: vertigo and nystagmus in the opposite direction from before, gradually fading away as the reflex adapts. But notice that the second bout of nystagmus, called Bechterew nystagmus,[38] is happening even though the labyrinths on both sides are gone. The slightly odd thing here is that if both labyrinths had been destroyed at the same time, there would have been no imbalance between right and left, and therefore no nystagmus. Bechterew nystagmus shows that the response to an injury depends on the organism's history, and that the brain contains at least a partial record of its previous adaptations, a chronicle of its past trials.[39]

Damage to the vestibulum has repercussions beyond the VOR: it also impairs the postural reflexes that control our trunk and limbs. That is why vestibular malfunctions can be detected by the senses of touch and joint position. For the VOR, though, the main measure of performance is visual; what matters is the stability of the retinal image.

Visual calibration

If you put on a pair of magnifying spectacles, your VOR is suddenly too weak. Suppose the glasses double the apparent size of everything you see; now when you turn your head to the left at 100 degrees per second, the visual world streams to the right at 200 degrees per second. To stabilize your retinal images, your VOR would have to rotate your eyes to the right at 200 degrees per second, which is double its usual response to that head motion. As soon as you put on the glasses and start moving around, your VOR will be somewhat augmented by visual tracking: you lock on to objects visually and track them with your eyes. But as we have seen, visual tracking can't cope with quick movements, so you will have many of the same problems as the physician whose labyrinths were poisoned with strep-tomycin. If you wear the glasses for a few hours, though, your performance will gradually improve. Furthermore—and this is the crucial point—the VOR remains abnormally strong even when tested in the dark.[40] It shrinks back to its former strength only gradually when the goggles are removed and normal vision is restored. In other words, altered vision can alter the oper-ation of the VOR.

This is a good thing, because the whole point of the VOR is to keep the retinal images stable. The bottom line is retinal slip: if the retinal images are fixed and clear, then the VOR is working properly; if the retinal images slip during head motion, then the VOR is improperly calibrated. The goggle experiment shows that the VOR is an adaptive network driven by an error signal coding retinal slip, or some closely related visual variable.

Different visual distortions induce different adaptations. Minifying specta-cles weaken the VOR. Reversing spectacles can even reverse it, so that the eyes move rightward when the head moves right.[41] Stranger adaptations can be evoked by computerized visual displays. These displays can, for instance, rotate the visual world upward whenever the head turns to the right; after a little of this, people develop a vertical eye rotation during horizontal head motion in darkness.[42]

How can the VOR strengthen or weaken itself? One option might be to strengthen or weaken the connections between motor neurons and eye muscles, but this would have unwanted side-effects, altering all sorts of eye movements which don't need adjustment because they are driven by vision, not by the vestibulum. For instance saccades, the quick move-ments which snap the eye from one visual target to another, can be visu-ally driven, so they can respond appropriately to visual targets even in the presence of distorting lenses. Seen through magnifying goggles, two targets that are in reality 10 degrees apart from the vantage point of the eye might appear 20 degrees apart. The result would be a saccade of 20 degrees rather than 10, but 20 degrees is just what you need to look from one target to the other through the goggles. In other words the saccadic system still makes accurate movements to visual targets, and needs no adaptation (though its response to auditory targets would have to be adjusted). That explains why no major changes are seen in the visually guided saccades of humans or animals adapting to magnifying spectacles. Evidently the diagnostic routines in the brain notice that sac-cades and other visually driven eye movements are normal, and so the malfunction in the VOR can't be due to a problem in the eye muscles. In the case of unilateral labyrinthine lesions, there is also little change in saccades during adaptation, presumably because the brain notices that they are normal whereas all vestibular reflexes are malfunctioning, and so, again, the problem can't be in the eye muscles. But how can a network of cells diagnose and repair itself? More generally, how can it reorganize itself to improve its performance, or in other words learn?

Machinery of learning

Simulated neural networks, running in computers, have learned to diagnose human diseases, to recognize vehicles from aerial photographs, and to detect bombs in x-ray pictures of airplane luggage. Their learning differs in some ways from what goes on in real neurons, but by studying it we can identify the issues and options facing all learning networks, including the brain.

I will talk about networks in terms of the operations they perform, converting their inputs into some sort of output. Many discussions of networks focus instead on their ability to recognize or remember patterns of input, but these are just special cases of the operator viewpoint. A pattern recognizer, for instance, is simply a network that performs a particular operation, receiving sensory data and producing distinct and consistent outputs in response to distinct patterns of input. This view of networks as operators rather than just recognizers or rememberers accords with one of the themes of this book, that the whole purpose of the brain is to perform sensorimotor transformations. Recognizing or remembering things contributes to our genetic success only in so far as it helps drive appropriate motor activity.

To learn is to rearrange your own brain in a way that improves your sensorimotor performance. When you learn to ride a bike, your brain modifies its own synapses (and probably other parts) to yield the right patterns of body motion in the right sensory contexts. Of course some learning isn't tied to any particular kind of sensory input or motor output. Having learned that the number of the planets is nine, I can take questions on that topic posed in various sensory forms, orally or in writing or maybe in gestures. And I can answer by various motor acts, by saying 'nine', by holding up nine fingers, by stamping my foot nine times like a counting horse, and so on. But this flexibility doesn't alter the fact that the learning was a change in my sensorimotor performance. In a simulated neural network, we usually designate some of the cells as input neurons, corresponding to the sense organs of the real brain, and some of the rest as output neurons, whose firing rates correspond to motor output. The network modifies its synapses in a way that changes its input–output relations. But how is this purposeful modification possible for a mere network of simple neurons?

Learning in a tiny brain

For the simplest possible illustration of learning, imagine a network with just one synapse. Its single neuron receives a single input which is amplified by the one synapse, so that if the input is 10 and the synaptic strength is 0.5, then the neuron's output, or in other words its firing rate, will be 5. For simplicity we will assume for now that the neuron performs no other processing. In particular its output doesn't saturate at any minimum or maximum firing rate, as would a real neuron's; its output is simply 0.5 times its input, however large or small that input may be. Now suppose we want this single-cell network to perform some operation, say doubling its inputs, so that an input of 10 yields an output of 20. We present the network with a series of inputs, say 1, 2, 3, and so on. For each input we compare the cell's output with the desired output, subtracting the actual from the desired. We will assume that the network starts out with a synaptic strength of 0.5. So if the input is 4, the desired output is 8 and the actual output is 2, giving an error of $8 - 2 = 6$. A positive error means that the synapse is too weak, while a negative error means that it is too strong. A simple learning mechanism would just strengthen the synapse a little after every positive error and weaken it after every negative error, adjusting it in this way until the outputs come to match the desired values, or in other words until the error becomes zero. In this simple case, all the errors will be positive at first, so the synapse will grow steadily stronger until it reaches its ideal value of 2, at which point the performance of the network on its doubling task will be perfect, the errors will all be zero, and the synapse will cease to change. In effect, the set of inputs and desired outputs, called the training set, provides the network with plenty of examples of what it is supposed to do, and the errors give it feedback about its performance. (Where do these error signals came from, in the brain? I will discuss this later in the chapter.)

In most cases, neural networks don't learn their operations well enough to drive the errors down to zero. For example, we can ask our monosynaptic network to perform a different transformation, a quadratic operation that turns the input x into the output $10x - x^2/20$. The graph of this operation is a curved line, so it must lie for ever beyond the reach of our poor, one-synapse network, which can never do anything other than multiply its input by a number, yielding a straight-line graph. It may adjust its synapse all it wants, but it will never be able to raise an input to the second power or subtract it from $10x$; it will never be able to generate any kind of curve. None the less, if we let the network learn as before, comparing actual with desired outputs, strengthening its synapse when the error is positive, weakening it when the error is negative, it will yield a better and better straight-line approximation to the unattainable curve. Eventually the network will have tuned itself to do the best job it can, reducing the error to the lowest attainable value, though that value will be greater than zero. Any further adjustment of the synapses may shrink the error for certain inputs, but will cause a larger increase in the error for other inputs. The optimal balance has been learned.

Energy landscapes

A useful way to think about learning involves what is called an energy landscape. Suppose we give our network a large batch of inputs, say all the whole numbers from 0 to 100. For each of these 101 inputs, the network will make an error; if it has learned its job perfectly, each error will be zero; otherwise, the errors will be non-zero. To measure the overall performance of the network, we might think of summing together all the errors for the individual inputs in the whole batch. But that won't work; a sum can be misleading because certain of the individual errors may be positive and others may be negative; these negatives and positives may cancel each other out in the sum, making it appear as though the network's performance is very good when in fact it is miserable. They may even sum precisely to zero, falsely suggesting perfect performance. To avoid this problem, the usual solution is to square all the errors before summing them; as both positive and negative errors yield positive numbers when squared, the sum of squared errors will be greater than zero unless all the individual errors are zero. So the sum of squared errors accurately reflects the network's performance. We call this sum of squares the cumulative error, or sometimes the cost or the energy function, because the network's goal is to make it as small as possible.

The cumulative error depends on the operation that our network is trying to learn, and on the current strength of its one synapse. For the doubling task, the optimal synaptic strength was 2, which yields an error of zero. What is the error when the synaptic strength is suboptimal, say equal to 1? Assuming, still, that the cumulative error is the sum of squared individual errors over all inputs from 0 to 100, the total comes to 338 350. If we plot a graph of cumulative error versus synaptic strength, we get a parabolic curve, touching zero where the synaptic strength equals 2 and rising steeply and endlessly on either side. It is helpful to regard this parabola as a two-dimensional, steep-sided valley with its deepest point at altitude zero. We call the parabola the error landscape of the network for this task, or more commonly the energy landscape, the idea being that the network is like a physical system that seeks its lowest energy level. From this perspective, the goal of learning is to reach the lowest spot in the energy landscape, or in other words to find the synaptic strength for which the cumulative error is smallest.

Learning can also be driven by 'success' rather than error signals, in which case the network should evolve so as to maximize cumulative success. Or there can be driving signals that move neither down to a minimum nor up to a maximum, but toward some other desired level. But in all cases the principles are analogous, so for definiteness I will continue to talk about error-driven learning and the search for deep spots in the energy landscape.

If we change the task, the energy landscape throws itself into a new form. For our quadratic task, computing $10x - x^2/20$, the landscape descends nowhere close to zero, but reaches a deepest level of about 320 325 where the synaptic strength is near 6.231. But the landscape is still a parabola whose smooth sides rise on either side of this minimum.

If we leave the task the same but change the training set, again the earth moves in the energy landscape. For example, if the network is still trying to learn the quadratic operation but the inputs in its training set now run from 50 to 150 instead of 0 to 100, the landscape reaches a deepest level of about 1 802 026 where the synaptic strength is about 4.217. This makes sense, because now we are asking the network to approximate a different portion of the quadratic curve, and so naturally it chooses a different straight line, with a different slope. So, in general, the energy landscape and therefore the final state of the synapse depend on the range of inputs to which the network is exposed. The same principle holds for the brain, and explains why any real sensorimotor system usually performs beautifully over its normal operating range but falls away badly from the optimum when its inputs stray outside that range.

Even with the shifted input range, though, the energy landscape of our monosynaptic network remains a parabola. Remarkably, the energy landscape for this network is always parabolic—sometimes broader, sometimes higher, but always a parabola. No matter how complex an operation the network is trying to learn, no matter what the range of inputs in its training set, its energy landscape always belongs to that same simple family of shapes. This same constancy holds for some, but by no means all, more complex networks. I will return to this point later.

Universal approximation

Most networks contain more than one cell, because large groups of cells can do things that single cells can't. That sounds obvious, but actually it is true only for certain types of cells. The lone neuron in our monosynaptic network, for instance, would benefit not at all from having more copies of itself around. Imagine, for instance, that the cell fed into another one like itself. If the first cell's synapse were of strength 2, say, it would amplify its inputs twofold. If the next cell's synapse were of strength 3, it would amplify its inputs threefold. So the net effect of the two cells in series would be to amplify the original input sixfold. But we could do that just as well using a single cell with a synapse of strength 6, unless for some reason synapses that powerful were ruled out. Until we hit the limit of the amplifying power of individual synapses, there is no functional advantage whatever to stringing two of these cells together in series. Cells like this are incapable of teamwork, so they would be poor raw material for a brain.[43]

This same limitation also holds for more complex cells with multiple input lines, as long as the cells are linear in the sense defined in Chapter 3 or in the Glossary (when the cell's inputs all double, for instance, its output doubles). No combination of linear cells, however large and intricate, can ever perform anything but linear computations, and that is a severe restriction because most mathematically possible computations, and most of the ones needed in a viable brain, are nonlinear. This is why I said in Chapter 3 that we could not survive with linear brains. In most simulated neural networks, and in the brain, the neurons are nonlinear.

The most popular type of nonlinear cell in simulated networks is the sigmoid neuron. As I said earlier, each such neuron receives a set of synaptic inputs which it multiplies by numbers called weights. The sum of all these weighted signals then represents the voltage across the cell membrane that determines its firing rate. But the cell's firing rate isn't precisely equal to this sum; across a middle range of voltages they rise together, but at very low and very high voltages the firing reaches its limits, never falling below zero and never rising above some maximum. A graph of firing rate versus voltage is roughly S-shaped, flattening out gradually at its upper and lower ranges and sloping steadily upward between the two. The S shape is used in part to make the network look more biological, because many real neurons show roughly this relation between input and firing. More importantly, though, the sigmoid nonlinearity makes the network versatile. Without the sigmoid function, the neurons would all be linear operators, and would be unable ever to achieve anything besides linear operations. But networks of sigmoid units can carry out any operation whatever, linear or nonlinear. A network of sigmoid neurons is a universal approximator in the sense that, given enough cells, it can closely match any operation, or at least any operation apart from bizarre, delicate ones that would occur only to a mathematician and that are unlikely to play any role in sensorimotor systems. There is nothing very special about sigmoid neurons, though. Universal approximation can be achieved with many types of nonlinear cell.[44]

Polysynaptic learning

How does a polysynaptic network learn? The procedure is much the same as with our monosynaptic network. Given an operation we want the network to perform, we provide it with many examples of the desired behavior. If we want it to add together two numbers, for instance, we feed the network's sensory, or input, neurons many pairs of addends. We want the firing rate of one cell, the output neuron, to equal the sum of the two inputs. Pairs of addends arrive one after the other, and for each pair the network yields an output. At each round, we compare this output with the desired value, namely the sum of the inputs, subtracting the actual output from the desired output to yield the error. If the network is doing its job perfectly, the error will be zero. If the network is imperfect, the error will provide a measure of its imperfection. Over a long run of many different inputs, the cumulative error or cost is the sum of all the individual squared errors.

As in the monosynaptic example, I will assume that learning proceeds by altering only the strengths of synapses, not any other network properties. The overall architecture of the network—which neurons are connected to which, and whether they are arrayed hierarchically in layers or cyclically in loops—I will assume to be hard-wired and unalterable. Similarly, neuron properties such as membrane permeabilities remote from the synapses I will assume remain fixed during learning. These assumptions are likely false, but I am making them only for the sake of concreteness, so that I can talk about synapses rather than a host of vaguely defined parameters. The principles of learning are much the same in any case; more generally, I would simply speak of altering network parameters instead of just synapses, of searching energy landscapes over parameter space instead of over synaptic space.

As in the monosynaptic case, the energy landscape is a graph of the network's error—its cumulative error in performing its task over a long series of inputs—as a function of its synaptic strengths. In the monosynaptic example the landscape was a two-dimensional graph of error versus the strength of the one synapse. When we are dealing with a large number, n, of synapses we can regard any set of synaptic strengths as a point in an n-dimensional realm called synaptic space. The idea, again, is to find the locus in synaptic space that yields the best-performing network. The energy landscape becomes an $n + 1$-dimensional graph, a hyperspace terrain where one dimension represents the height of the land—the cumulative error—and the other n dimensions represent the strengths of all the synapses. This notion of a hyperdimensional landscape can help us understand learning. It might not seem that way at first glance, given that we can't easily picture hyperdimensional scenes. But with mathematics we can calculate our way through hyperspace. As far as intuition goes, the idea is to picture the energy landscape as three-dimensional, so as to get a feel for the principles that also apply in higher dimensions.

For some synaptic strengths, the network's cumulative error is small, maybe even zero; these are the coveted low spots in the energy landscape. For other synaptic strengths (that is for other points in synaptic space), the cumulative error rises very high, forming a hill. As before, we can picture learning as a search for low spots, valleys and basins among the hills of the energy landscape (and also as before, the same principles govern success-driven learning, which seeks out high rather than low points in the landscape).

The only real difference from the monosynaptic case is that in a polysynaptic network it is harder to work out, based on the error signals, whether any given synapse should be strengthened or weakened and by how much, because the ideal adjustment to any one synapse depends on what all the other synapses are doing. Ideally, then, the learning mechanism must gather information from the whole network and bring it to bear on each synapse.

Another way to put this is that a polysynaptic network can have a more complex energy landscape. In our monosynaptic example, the landscape was just a parabola. To learn was simply to adjust our synapse toward the bottom of the parabola rather than away from it, and to keep stepping in that same direction until the minimum was reached. It is a greater challenge to navigate a hyperdimensional landscape, which can be a wildly complicated terrain of hills and basins, ridges, and twisting valleys.

And the landscape metaphor can actually make the task sound easier than it really is. If we were standing in hilly terrain, searching for the deepest spot, we would start by looking around, scanning for low places. But a learning network can't 'scan' the energy landscape. It has to compute how its performance would change if it were to adopt some new set of synaptic strengths. The computations may be slow, and generally have to be done for one candidate set of synaptic strengths at a time. We get a better feel for the problem if we imagine ourselves standing on a slope in the energy landscape in pitch darkness, our way lit only by a pencil-beamed flashlight—a cumbersome flashlight that we can redirect only slowly.

Ideally, we want to find the deepest point in the energy landscape, the global optimum, where the error is smallest, but often this goal is out of reach. Finding the global optimum amidst all the complexity of the energy landscape is usually not feasible, so we settle instead for some low basin, deeper than any of the immediately surrounding countryside, but not necessarily as deep as the global optimum. These basins are called local optima, and often they are good enough. With these synaptic settings, the network may perform its operation tolerably well.

Mathematicians were searching energy landscapes for optima, global and local, long before the advent of simulated neural networks. This is the mathematical problem of optimization, which has endless applications in science and industry. So learning is a special case of optimization, and most of the many algorithms developed for optimization translate into mechanisms for learning. Of all optimization techniques the most powerful and versatile is the method of gradient descent, whose closest counterpart in learning theory is called back-propagation, or backprop.[45, 46]

Slippery slope

The backprop algorithm makes repeated, small adjustments to all the synapses of the network, each change slightly improving the network's performance. It tries to make each change as efficacious as possible, to yield the biggest reduction in cumulative error that is possible with a synaptic adjustment of that size. The changes continue until the network shows no further improvement. The idea is that the network should move like a toboggan through the energy landscape, sliding down the slopes until it comes to rest in a deep hollow. The hollow may be a local rather than a global optimum, but again, a local optimum is often good enough.

How does the backprop algorithm compute the most efficacious adjustment to the synapses, or in other words the direction of steepest downward slope in the energy landscape? Computing the direction of steepest descent involves knowing something about every dimension of synaptic space: the algorithm modifies each synapse based on information gathered from all other synapses. There is no need here to go into the details of the computation, but as the name back-propagation suggests, it requires that the network transmit information about synaptic strengths backwards through the network, from downstream synapses to synapses further upstream.

Biological plausibility

Many neuroscientists feel that back-propagation is not a biologically plausible learning mechanism, though the arguments are not conclusive.

One perceived implausibility of backprop is that it transmits information backward across synapses and up axons toward cell bodies, whereas in reality action potentials flow along axons in only one direction, away from the cell body. But this is a weak objection. For one thing, the information could be carried backward by other axons running the other way. Or signals may run backwards across synapses and up axons after all. The fact that action potentials normally move down axons doesn't preclude other chemical processes carrying information the other way.[47] Indeed there is evidence for fairly rapid long-range intracellular signaling in the cytoplasm, and there are substances that pass backwards across synapses and could act as retrotransmitters,[48, 49] though there are questions as to whether this signaling could offer the temporal precision that is needed for backprop.

Another objection is that the backward-flowing signals must carry information about remote synapses, and how could one synapse be informed of another's properties, which depend on local concentrations of various molecules? In fact there are many ways this could be done—via other, back-projecting neurons or via retrotransmitters and cytoplasmic transport—and not all of these mechanisms can be dismissed out of hand.[50] Evidence from cell cultures suggests that synaptic information can propagate backwards.[51, 52] Given the advantages it would bring for learning, it is entirely plausible that neurons have evolved molecular machinery for transmitting data about synapses.

A third common complaint is that backprop networks supposedly cannot learn complex transformations. This charge is sometimes supported by citing a classic paper[53] by Stuart Geman, Elie Bienenstock, and René Doursat, but actually their findings in no way impugn backprop. They showed that extremely versatile networks, like those used in most backprop studies, need a lot of information to learn a pattern, whereas more specialized networks can learn with less. Their argument suggests that learning in the brain may start with congenitally specialized networks rather than absolutely general-purpose ones, but it implies nothing about backprop, which is just as useful for specialized networks as it is for more versatile ones.

But even if backprop is biologically feasible, it is admittedly elaborate, and a simpler option would be welcome. It seems likely that biological learning works by gradient descent, which is the most powerful optimization method ever discovered, but there are other ways, besides the standard back-propagation algorithm, of computing or approximating the direction of steepest descent in an energy landscape. So far, however, no one has found an alternative algorithm that is clearly more plausible biologically than backprop, yet matches its versatility and speed. And speed is a major concern, as even backprop sometimes appears to be an implausibly slow way to train networks containing thousands or millions of neurons.

Speed

Most people respond to the backprop algorithm in one of two ways. Neuroscientists tend to covet its beauty from afar, seeing it as wonderfully fast and efficient but sadly unbiological. Computer scientists, who don't much care about biology, consider standard, unadorned backprop dumpy and slow. Compared with most of the learning algorithms that are usually considered biologically plausible, backprop really is lightning-fast, but it is true that it can be greatly accelerated.

I said that backprop finds the direction of steepest descent in the energy landscape and then alters the synapses, shifting the network a small distance in that direction. Computing the steepest direction is easy, but finding the optimal distance is harder. In its simplest form, the backprop algorithm offers no recommendation at all about distance. It is up to the user to guess the optimal step size. If we choose small steps, the algorithm proceeds slowly, like a sticky toboggan lurching down a snow-free hill. We can hasten the descent by taking larger steps, but if the steps become too large they may overshoot the low ground and land higher rather than lower on the energy surface. The network moves through its landscape in an untoboggan-like way. At best, it looks like Wile E. Coyote on a toboggan: it zig-zags down gorges not by snaking along the bottom but by bouncing back and forth between the canyon walls. Make the steps just a little bit larger still, and it is easy to make the proceedings fly completely out of control: our toboggan is flung into remote, inhospitable corners of synaptic space where the errors are astronomical, and from which it takes a long time to find its way back.

One way to speed up the descent and avoid zig-zagging is to add momentum. This means that at each step in the algorithm instead of driving the toboggan exactly in the current direction of steepest descent, you drive it along a path that is a mix between the steepest slope and the direction of motion in the previous step. If backprop is like letting a sticky toboggan slide down a hill with a lot of friction, so that it always takes the steepest path, then backprop with momentum is like greasing the bottom, reducing the friction so that the toboggan can build up impetus. Then it is not so strongly deflected by small dips and slants in the landscape. Instead of zig-zagging with the local gradient, it tends to carry on in the general direction it has been moving. The result is a smoother path and a faster descent. And if synaptic information can travel cytoplasmically, as I suggested earlier, then backprop with momentum is as biologically plausible as backprop alone.

Still faster descent can be achieved by computing, at each step, not just the direction of steepest slope in the energy landscape but also its local curvature. With these data, the algorithm can pick an optimal step size in each round. Calculating curvature takes time in computer simulations, but if handled smartly it is worth it: all the fastest versions of backprop use information about the curvature of the energy landscape.[54] It remains to be seen whether the brain's learning algorithm does the same.

Even with these hot-rod accessories, the backprop algorithm can't usually find an optimum for a network of n synapses in fewer than n steps.[54] In a computer, each of the n steps requires at least $3n$ arithmetic operations— multiplications and additions. So the trip to the optimum involves a total of at least $3n \times n$, or $3n^2$ operations. Optimizing a network of 10 million synapses would take 300 trillion arithmetic calculations. It sounds as though we should be spectacularly, geologically slow on the uptake. Why doesn't it take us a million years to learn to tie our shoes? It is important to remember that in the brain multiple arithmetic operations can occur at the same time. A backprop network could theoretically be arranged so that each of the n synapses computes its own adjustments. That arrangement would speed things up n-fold. Further, it is in principle possible that the arithmetic operations performed by each of the n synapses at each of the n steps could occur in parallel, further accelerating the process. So the number of time steps needed to optimize an n-synapse network may be about n, which is still a lot, but better than $3n^2$.

Seeking the global optimum

Somewhere in the energy landscape is the ultimate prize, the King Solomon's mines of our story—the global optimum. But as I have said, it is usually out of reach. Backprop generally sticks in a local optimum rather than the global one. In a complex landscape this is almost always what happens. It is satisfactory if the local optimum is deep enough, but the global optimum would be better. Unfortunately, there is no tractable algorithm that is guaranteed to find global optima in arbitrary energy landscapes, and there probably never will be. The difficulty is that the global optimum could be anywhere; its basin could be tiny, shaped like a deep well, so that the local conditions even very close by might offer no clue that the optimum is near. Nevertheless, there are techniques that, in certain types of landscape, increase our chances of reaching the global optimum, or at least of avoiding shallow local optima and landing in deep ones. At present it is an open question whether biological learning does anything to avoid shallow local optima, but doing so might bring major advantages, and there are a number of ways it might be done.

One approach is just to run the backprop algorithm several times, starting from different points in the landscape, and keep track of which run gave the best result. Adding momentum will speed up each run, and in fact momentum itself can sometimes carry the network out of shallow dips into deeper basins. For this to work in the brain, synapses would need some way to store information about their former weights and the associated errors, so the network could try out various settings but still return to the best ones it had found so far.

Another method is to jump around randomly in synaptic space. After each jump, we measure the height of the landscape at our current location, always remembering which of the spots we have visited so far was the deepest. Continued long enough, this method is guaranteed to bring us to the global optimum, though we won't usually know when we have reached it, and in any case the process normally takes longer than the age of the universe. A faster variant called simulated annealing[55] combines steepest descent with a certain amount of random jittering around, so that sometimes it takes a step up rather than down the slope. Because we usually need a large upward movement, or a large number of small ones, to exit a deep basin, any one upward step is more likely to take the network out of a shallow basin than out of a deep one, so the method allows us to escape from poor minima into better ones. The process is slow, but then so are all methods of global optimization in complex landscapes.

A third way to search for global optima is the method of graduated non-convexity.[56] Here we start by approximating the energy landscape with a simpler one where the global optimum is easy to find. Once we have found it, we choose a new landscape, very much like our initial one but resembling slightly more closely the real, target landscape. We descend into the nearest local optimum of our new landscape, and hope that, because the new landscape isn't so very different from the old one, the local optimum we land in will still be the global optimum. Over many steps we introduce more and more complexity, gradually morphing our landscape into the one of interest, but hoping that the global optimum will stay in the same vicinity or will wander away only gradually, so that we can repeatedly descend back into it. If the problem is gradually elaborated in the right way, this method can sometimes guide us into the global optimum of the final, complex landscape. This sounds like a promising way to build a fetal or infant brain, but could this idea of gradual complication also be used to recalibrate mature brains? When a network began a phase of intensive learning (when it noticed that it had been making large errors) it might simplify its energy landscape, perhaps by restricting its task in some way, or by simplifying its own processing, for instance by supressing the nonlinearities in its neurons, and then gradually reintroduce complexity. I know of no evidence for any process like this in the brain, but it is possible.

Genetic algorithm

A fourth method of global optimization is the genetic algorithm.[57-59] In this approach, we think of each point in synaptic space—each possible set of synaptic strengths for the network—as being like a set of possible genes for an organism. The depth of the landscape at any point now represents the adaptive fitness of that set of genes, and the search for an optimum represents evolution toward the best genome. In the computer we randomly create several organisms with different genomes, check their fitness, and let the fittest among them 'mate', mixing their genes, in the hope that their offspring over many generations will evolve toward the global optimum.

Notice that this procedure, when we describe it in terms of the metaphor of toboggans and energy landscapes, doesn't at first seem promising: you place several toboggans at random points in the energy landscape, measure their altitudes, and then 'mate' the deepest ones by mixing their coordinates, for instance giving one baby toboggan the east–west location, or longitude, of one parent and the north–south location, or latitude, of another parent. Why should this mixing help? In most landscapes there is no reason to expect the baby toboggan to lie particularly deep. But then why does the same procedure make sense when expressed in terms of genes, and why does it often work in practice? The procedure works when fitness separates into independent factors, or 'modules'. Genetically, this may often be the case: if your mother has perfected the genome for eyes and your father has exquisite ears, then with luck you may inherit both advantages.

Can we understand the process in terms of the toboggan metaphor, which has elsewhere been so useful? In what sense might an energy landscape be 'modular'? One thing it might mean is that the contour along, say, the east–west dimension doesn't change its shape as we move north or south, though the whole rigid contour may rise or descend, and similarly for the north–south contour. Then if one toboggan is lying in a deep valley in the east–west dimension and another is doing the same in the north–south dimension, their baby toboggan has a fair chance of lying deeper than its parents, in the combined basin where the two valleys meet. (Of course in a strictly modular landscape of this sort we can often find the global optimum even without the genetic algorithm—just find the minimum for one dimension at a time. So what sorts of landscapes are specifically amenable to the genetic approach, more than to other optimization algorithms? That is not well understood.)

The brain might combine the genetic algorithm with back-propagation, setting several toboggans sliding downhill, repeatedly checking which are doing best—which have reached the deepest chasms—then mixing the locations of the best-placed toboggans and continuing the slides from the new sites. So the genetic algorithm, though it was designed to mimic natural selection, might also work in the brain.

Energy landscaping

There is another way to avoid bad local optima, and that is to arrange the energy landscape so that there are none. We give up trying to navigate complex energy landscapes and instead build our networks in such a way that their landscapes retain a simple shape even when they are multidimensional. In general, the shape of the energy landscape depends on the properties of the individual neurons in our network; on how the neurons are wired together, whether in a single layer, a series of many layers, or in loops; and on the operation we want the network to learn. But it is possible to organize the network so that, no matter what operation it is learning, its energy landscape is always simple, always a smooth-walled bowl with no plateaus or shallow basins to snag the toboggan. In this sort of landscape, backprop always takes us swiftly to the global optimum.

The way to guarantee bowl-shaped landscapes is to restrict learning to a set of simple output cells. In any network, some of the neurons receive the inputs to the network, others are interneurons, and some are the output cells, whose activities we want to be some functions of the inputs. I am now supposing that only the synapses on to these output cells are modifiable by learning—all the rest are fixed—and that the output neurons themselves are simple in this sense: their activity is just the sum of the signals coming through their synapses.

For a network like this, the energy landscape is always a smooth bowl, regardless of the task that is being learned. It is like the monosynaptic network at the start of the chapter, where the landscape was always a parabola, except that now it is a hyperdimensional paraboloid, its smooth walls all dropping down to the single, global optimum. Why is the landscape so simple? As usual, it describes how cumulative error rises and falls with the various possible strengths of the synapses, but now the only synapses under consideration are those in the output layer. No other neurons, no complex transformations, intervene between the modifiable synapses and the output of the whole network, so the relation between synaptic strength and error is unusually simple. In any such network, there is no danger of sticking anywhere but the global optimum.

Another advantage of output-layer learning is that the network can store past experience and use it to guide learning in the present. The learning equations for these networks are such that the adjustable parameters—the strengths of the modifiable synapses—can be isolated from the terms representing sensory input and error. It takes some algebra to prove it, but the result is that the sensory data and error signals experienced by the network over any span of time can be gathered and stored in a mathematically convenient representation, which can be used to guide learning (in fact the storage space you need doesn't increase with the duration of the experience being stored—a day takes up no more space than a minute). So this sort of network could adjust its synapses now, based on experience collected in the past. It could improve its skating technique by sitting in an armchair in the evening and mulling over its afternoon spent staggering around on the rink. But this works *only* for a single layer of adaptable synapses. In other architectures, the learning equations don't isolate the parameters in the same way, so the network can't so conveniently use past experience to guide present learning. Whether the real brain is capable of doing this is another open question.

Output-layer learning can support remarkably lifelike behavior. The most impressive example I know is Murphy, who is a robot designed by Bartlett W. Mel and engagingly described in Mel's 1990 book *Connectionist Robot Motion Planning.*[60] Murphy has a single camera eye poised above a tabletop and looking down at it. He has a three-jointed arm that bends in the plane of the table, and a brain in which single layers of teachable synapses learn to move his hand toward visual targets. With the help of these synapses, Murphy can mentally rehearse tricky arm motions before executing them. He can plan complex movements that let him snake his arm around the obstacles in his path. Reading of his adventures in Mel's book, I became a fan of Murphy; I would like to see further stories about him, though maybe this time with a love interest and some more exotic locales.

If output-layer learning lets us practice skating in an armchair, if it delivers us to the global optimum for any task, why does anyone ever bother with other kinds of learning? The weakness of output-layer learning is that it loses flexibility because none of the synapses outside that layer can learn. At the beginning of the game, you guess what synaptic strengths you might need in the interior of your network, and then you have to live with them. Faced with any task, you quickly descend into the global optimum of the energy landscape; in other words you learn to do the task as well as it can be done, given the frozen synapses you have chosen, but more than likely, if those synapses were unfrozen and allowed to learn, you could do the job even better. Another way to put this is that arriving at the global optimum isn't necessarily a triumph unless that optimum is a deep one. It is better to halt in a deep local optimum of a complex landscape than in the shallow global optimum of a simple landscape. So networks with just one layer of learning have smooth energy surfaces, but in return they have to accept a rigid structure which reduces their versatility.

But then again, if we have enough interior neurons, and if we set their unteachable synapses so that they perform a wide variety of operations, might we not have the resources to learn any task that comes along? I can entertain a vision of the brain that works this way, where all the learning is confined to a single output layer, driven by a vast array of frozen, almost infinitely varied, nonlinear operators—a thin shell of learning on an amorphous interior of general-purpose transformations, like chocolate surrounding a fondant filling.

Actually, the interior would be less like fondant filling than like a universal toolbox. Every interior neuron is a tool that performs some operation on some set of inputs. Every tool can be made available to every sensorimotor system in the brain, simply by connecting that neuron to an output cell of that system. Sharing is not a problem. If different systems need the same tool simultaneously for different tasks, the same interior neuron can project to different output neurons, just as the network cells in Chapter 3 projected to two output cells, one for addition and one for multiplication. If a sensorimotor system has no need of a given tool, then its connection to that neuron is weakened or eliminated. In a rough way this picture fits what we know of brain development, where huge numbers of connections form in the fetal brain and are then drastically pruned. Maybe the pruning is the different sensorimotor systems sorting out which tools they need. On this view, your central toolbox contains every elementary concept you will ever have, and learning is a matter of combining these concepts into a useful vocabulary of thought and action.

In the end, the idea of a brain built entirely on output-layer learning still seems to me implausible. I am offended by the sheer wasted potential in those ranks upon ranks of stolid, unteachable synapses. More appealing would be a hybrid scheme, where the synapses in the output layer swiftly find their globally optimal settings while something like backprop more slowly improves that global optimum by adjusting the interior synapses. An important point here is that for output-layer as for backprop learning, the output cells of the learning network need not be the output cells of the brain as a whole, the motor neurons; they can be any cells for which it is possible to specify a desired output; that is, for which there is an error signal that gauges their performance in some useful way and can therefore drive learning. But I want to postpone this question of the brain's output layer to the end of Chapter 7, where I discuss learning through an interface.

Unsupervised learning

So far, the learning I have described has all been driven by error signals that compare their network's performance with some desired behavior; the point of the learning is to drive the error down as close as possible to zero. This is called supervised learning, the idea being that the error signal is checking and guiding the network's education. There is another sort of learning, called unsupervised, where there is no error signal.

Maybe the simplest example involves, again, a single neuron that receives a single input and amplifies it by some factor. The amplification factor depends on the strength of the cell's one synapse: if the input signal is 5 and the synaptic strength is 4, for instance, then the cell's output, or firing rate, is 4 times 5, or 20. Suppose that the synapse is so constituted that it automatically adjusts itself to match its input. If the input is steady at 5, then the synapse gradually adjusts itself until it equilibrates at 5, giving an output of 5 times 5, or 25. If the input is steady at 3, the synapse adapts until its value is 3, giving an output of 9. Given any steady input, then, this cell learns to square it. And it learns this with no help from any error signal. This particular example may not be inspiring, but unsupervised networks, cunningly arranged, can achieve remarkable things. Teuvo Kohonen, for instance, has shown how simple unsupervised networks, driven by retinal cells, can organize themselves into maps of visual space like those in the superior colliculus and visual cortex.[61]

Most networks in the brain are probably the end products of genetic hard-wiring, unsupervised learning, and error-driven supervised learning. They can't survive on hard-wiring and unsupervised learning alone, because in a sensorimotor system what matters is motor performance. If the network had no error signal to tell it how well it was doing its job, if it were driving blind, then it would stray into confusion. If a malfunction elsewhere in the brain, or in the bones or muscles, affected its performance, the network would never learn about it. It needs a signal that conveys the bottom line, an error signal coding some sensory measure of the system's overall performance.

The brain's repair shop

Maybe the best-studied example of error-driven learning is the adaptation of the VOR, which is driven by signals coding retinal slip. Despite all the study, we are still unsure how visual signals alter the synapses of the VOR, but we know that a crucial role is played by the cerebellum, which D. A. Robinson called the repair shop of the brain.

Cerebellum is Latin for little brain. The name was meant to distinguish it from the big brain, the cerebral hemispheres, though the outer rind, or cortex, of the cerebellum contains some 70 billion neurons, apparently more than the whole cerebral cortex.[62] The cerebellum sits tucked under the back of the cerebrum and on top of the brainstem.

Damage to the cerebellum causes a wide range of deficits, including clumsiness, tremor, slurred speech, unsteady gait, and impaired timing and time perception. The same problems are seen in drunkenness, because alcohol has a potent effect on the cerebellum (this is not to say that all features of inebriation are cerebellar—cerebellar disease doesn't make you dance around with a lampshade on your head). Many of these deficits may arise because patients (and drinkers) lose patterns of coordination that have been learned and stored in the cerebellum.

We know that the cerebellum plays a role in adaptation. Lesions impair motor learning, and lesions to different areas impair it in different ways, some blocking VOR adaptation, others making it impossible to re-establish accurate gaze shifts after the eye muscles are weakened.[63-65] Cerebellar lesions can also erase previous adaptations. This shows us that, at least in some cases, the cerebellum doesn't act like a TV repairperson, stepping in to fix malfunctioning circuits and then leaving things to run on their own. Instead, the cerebellum seems to have ongoing responsibilities, maintaining the repaired circuits. The altered circuits may themselves be in the cerebellum, or they may be elsewhere.

Wiring

All 70 billion neurons in the cerebellar cortex are wired together in a uniform pattern.[1] The sole output cells of this array are the large neurons called Purkinje cells, which are inhibitory, meaning that they suppress activity in the neurons they project to. It may seem odd that the only command ever issued by this prodigious network is 'quieten down', but many of the neurons that the Purkinje cells inhibit are themselves inhibitory neurons, whose suppression disinhibits neurons further downstream. So the net effect of a command from the cerebellum is a complex downstream pattern of inhibition and excitation.

Two main inputs reach the cerebellum: the mossy fibers, which arise from many places in the brain and spinal cord, and the climbing fibers, which all arise from a single small node, the inferior olivary nucleus. Mossy fibers influence thousands of Purkinje cells, though they do it indirectly. Inside the cerebellar cortex they excite neurons called granule cells. Granule-cell axons, known as parallel fibers, run like billions of telephone wires just beneath the cortical surface. The parallel fibers contact Purkinje cells directly and via inhibitory neurons. Each Purkinje cell is contacted by up to 200 000 parallel fibers. Together, these thousands of fibers evoke in the Purkinje cell about 100 responses, called simple spikes, every second. Each climbing fiber, on the other hand, contacts only about ten Purkinje cells, and each Purkinje cell receives synapses from just one climbing fiber. These fibers carry signals, or action potentials, at an average rate of about one per second, each potential eliciting in each of its target Purkinje cells a rapid cluster of activity called a complex spike. What is the purpose of this arrangement?

Marr and Albus

In 1969, David Marr suggested that the cerebellar cortex is a machine for learning sensorimotor tasks.[66] He proposed that the modifiable synapses are those between the parallel fibers and the Purkinje cells. Climbing fibers carry the error signals that drive learning. Parallel fibers supply a huge and continuous flood of diverse signals—visual, auditory, tactile, vestibular, proprioceptive, motor, cognitive. These signals provide raw material for a huge range of sensorimotor transformations. They are like the universal toolbox I described earlier in the context of output-layer learning.

Marr proposed that the synapse between a parallel fiber and a Purkinje cell strengthens whenever the fiber and the cell both fire at the same time. When teaching signals from a climbing fiber repeatedly cause a Purkinje cell to fire during a particular pattern of parallel-fiber activity, the synaptic connections strengthen until those parallel fibers are able to fire the Purkinje cell all by themselves, without help from the climbing fiber. In a variant of the theory, proposed by James Albus in 1971, the synapses don't strengthen but weaken with simultaneous firing.[67] Albus's version appears to fit the physiology better,[68, 69] but it doesn't alter the basic idea of the theory—it relates to Marr's version somewhat as a developed picture relates to a photographic negative.

Some aspects of the Marr–Albus theory have empirical support. As the theory predicts, lesions to the cerebellum or inferior olive can prevent adaptation.[70-73] Further, climbing fibers are unusually active during learning, and their influence causes enduring changes in the synapses joining parallel fibers and Purkinje cells.[72, 74]

Masao Ito and others have shown that the Marr–Albus scheme can explain some aspects of adaptation in the VOR.[72] Some Purkinje cells receive parallel fibers carrying head-velocity signals from the inner ear, and it is likely that these same cells project to secondary vestibular neurons, so they are well placed to influence the VOR. These Purkinje cells also appear to receive, from climbing fibers, an error signal coding the slip velocity of the retinal images. If the VOR is working perfectly then there is no retinal slip and these climbing fibers are silent. But if minifying spectacles are placed before your eyes, the climbing fibers carry a retinal-slip signal.

Now all the pieces are in place for learning: every time you turn your head, the parallel fiber and the climbing fiber both excite the Purkinje cell. As a result the synapse from the parallel fiber to the Purkinje cell changes, strengthening in Marr's version, weakening in Albus's. Altered Purkinje activity affects the secondary vestibular neuron, so that neuron transmits an altered eye-velocity command to the motor neurons. In this way the VOR is adjusted. As adaptation proceeds, the activity in the climbing fiber declines, but the modified synapse on the Purkinje cell retains its changes, so the VOR will remain adapted until you take off the minifying spectacles and start to drive the adaptation back the other way.

But Stephen Lisberger and others have shown that the Marr–Albus model will have to be extended to fit certain aspects of learning in the VOR. They have shown for instance that other synapses besides those between parallel fibers and Purkinje cells, specifically synapses in the vestibular nuclei, are plastic and contribute to learning.[75]

The VOR is a relatively simple example, but the Marr–Albus mechanism can learn arbitrarily complex transformations. It can also explain the automation of motor patterns with practice. When you learn to play a tune on the piano you first consciously direct each finger placement, but after some practice you need only consciously start the piece and the rest flows automatically. The Marr–Albus model can do the same thing: after a little practice, the pattern of sound, touch, and body sense from each key-press, conveyed by parallel fibers, automatically triggers the Purkinje cells that order the next key press. Computer programs based on the Marr–Albus mechanism are capable of learning huge numbers of motor sequences and have been used to train robots.

The Marr–Albus scheme is an example of output-layer learning. It involves no complex backprop, but merely conveys an error message to a single layer of modifiable synapses between parallel fibers and Purkinje cells. The Purkinje cells are not the output cells for any sensorimotor sys-tem, because they don't contact the muscles directly, but as I have said, they can still be the output cells of a learning network, as long as there exists an error signal for them: a signal that gauges their deviations from some desired pattern of activity. In the theory the error signals are carried by the climbing fibers, all of which arise from the inferior olivary nucleus, so it is the cells in the inferior olive that know what every Purkinje cell should be doing, though how they know it is not yet clear.

How learning could simplify the genome

At the start of this chapter I said that learning lets an organism cope with uncertainty, including uncertainty within its own body: as you can't know beforehand the exact mechanical properties of your vestibular sensors or your eye muscles, you need a VOR that can adapt to whatever it finds. Learning has other functions as well; for instance it can speed up evolu-tion by the 'Baldwin effect'.[76, 77] Here I will argue that learning is also one way to zip the brain: to simplify the genetic instructions for building it. For instance, it may be possible to compress the genomic code for the VOR by coding not a finished reflex but a learning network that shapes itself into a VOR based on sensory information. But why should this be true? Why should you need a smaller genome to code a protoreflex than a finished reflex?

The reason may seem obvious if you think of a learning network as drawing information out of the environment, as a life-raft inflates itself by sucking air out of its surroundings. Clearly, it might seem, if some of the information in the finished network is coming from the environment, then you need less of it in the genome. But this is no argument, because 'drawing information out of the environment' is a complex matter, requir-ing intricate machinery that has to be coded genetically. The real question is, will it be simpler to code the learning machinery than to code the finished network? Is there any reason to think it is simpler to code in the genome an adaptive network that forms itself into a sensorimotor system than it would be just to code, quite straightforwardly, the connections you want between the sensors and muscles?

Mathematically, there is. First of all, it is plausible that the learning machinery is largely alike throughout the brain, or over large portions of the brain, because a single learning mechanism can learn a huge range of different operations. Theoretically, every sensorimotor system in the brain might work on just one learning mechanism, for instance the cytoplasmic backprop that I mentioned earlier. If this is true in the brain, or even if the brain works on a small handful of basic algorithms, then the learning machinery could be the same for vast numbers of neurons. In the genome it could be coded just once in the basic recipe for those neurons, along with membranes and synapses and the other apparatus that is common to all the cells in the group.

If the learning machinery is largely uniform, then the differences between different networks lie in their inputs and outputs—their sense organs and muscles—and in their size and wiring patterns, and, most crucially, in the error signals that determine what they learn. All of this would have to be specified genetically. The error signals would have to be computed by some network from sense inputs of its own, which may well be different from the inputs to the sensorimotor system it is teaching. For example the VOR is driven by vestibular inputs, but it is taught by retinal-slip information gathered by the eyes. The error-computing network would either have to be genetically specified in all its finished detail, or it would have to form itself by learning, perhaps involving error-driven, supervised learning, in which case the error signals for that learning would have to come from a third network. Eventually, we will reach bedrock, arriving at some error-computing network that has to be specified genetically. So the argument that learning can simplify the genome comes down to the claim that it is simpler to build a network that computes an error signal than to build the finished network we really want, which computes some useful sensorimotor transformation. Why should this be so?

No mathematical rule says that the error signal for a learning network has to be easier to compute than the operation the network is trying to learn. It is entirely possible to use a complex error signal to teach a network a simple operation. But there is a potentially useful asymmetry here: for any operation that you want a network to learn, there is an infinity of different error signals that could teach it. Many of these will be *more* complex to compute than the function that you want the network to learn. But just because there are so many different error signals, there is a chance that one or two among them will be simpler to compute than the network operation. And some error signals may come for free, in the sense that we need them anyway for other purposes, so it costs nothing extra to make them available for learning. For example, the retinal-slip signals that shape the VOR would likely exist anyway, even if there were no VOR, because we need them to sense visual motion. So the VOR shares the cost of its error signal with the visual system. Natural selection could seek out these kinds of simple, shared, or pre-existing error signals, which would simplify the genomic code for the brain.

Understanding adaptive networks

Everyone agrees that the brain is a giant network of neurons, but many scientists believe that neural network concepts alone won't enable us to comprehend the brain.[6] Instead we need 'higher-level' concepts, maybe more psychological ones, maybe involving the idea of a symbol. I am sure it is true that useful new concepts will emerge with time, and I can't imagine what fundamental concepts may underlie neuroscience a century from now, but I am suggesting that we can go a long way toward understanding real neuronal networks using the concept of self-optimization.

It is usually impossible to apprehend in detail how a network of any complexity does its job, but if the network is shaped by supervised learning we can often achieve a perfectly satisfactory understanding of it by answering two questions: what is the learning algorithm and what are the signals—the errors or successes—that drive its adaptation? If we know these things, we can build functionally equivalent networks by computer simulation. Of the two questions, the second is often more important in deciphering the network's function. In flexible, versatile learning networks it is the error or success signals that largely determine the operation of the finished network. Change them, and you usually change the performance. The learning mechanism matters less because it can vary greatly without much affecting the final outcome. Entirely different network architectures, made of different types of cells and using different learning rules, will all come to do about the same job if they are driven by the same signals. In less versatile, more specialized networks, where supervised learning is limited to mere fine-tuning, the error signals may not be so revealing, but still they give useful clues to the network's construction. If you can ask only one question about the inner workings of a supervised learning network, and that means practically any sensorimotor network in the brain, the question should probably be, 'What are the signals that drive learning?'

The program

Our aim is a rigorous understanding of the brain, meaning one whose concepts can be analyzed down to the level of pure logic and programmed on a computer. To cope with the brain's complexity, we seek principles of order within it. The example of the egg cell suggests that this search is likely to pay off: the brain is highly ordered, and can be simplified dramatically by exploiting that fact. Finding the order in the brain may be a challenge, but at least we can be confident that it is there.

A crucial clue is that the brain was created by natural selection, which is an optimizing process. What it optimizes is the brain's sensorimotor performance, so we can gain insight into real brains by considering how an optimal brain would behave. Probably the most powerful optimizing mechanism ever invented by natural selection was learning, so we should look for sensorimotor optimization principles that could be learned based on signals from our sense organs. If we know the optimization principles we can draw out their logical implications with computers. Among other uses, computer simulations may help us deduce the microscopic workings of the brain—knowing what the networks are doing may help us understand their details. But even if a neuron-by-neuron account of the brain is for ever out of reach, still the program of identifying the optimization principles that shape the brain is in itself a useful, feasible, and inspiring goal.

Many optimization principles will be easier to deduce from the behavior of the whole organism than from samples of neuronal activity, that is by a sort of aerial survey rather than by cutting through the jungle. In the following chapters I will pursue this program in a number of simple systems, exploring different aspects of neural optimization.

Chapter 6

Unfolding in time

In the 17th century, Johannes Kepler, Isaac Newton, and others made the momentous discovery that many aspects of order in the universe, including some of the most basic laws of nature, can't be seen in a single snapshot but are manifest in the way things unfold in time. Nature's patterns are temporal patterns. To survive in this dynamic universe, the brain has to be able to detect and create order in temporal streams of signals.

Most of what the brain does, from vision to speech comprehension to steering the eyes and limbs, involves sensing and controlling temporal patterns. Music, for instance, affects our brains largely through its temporal unfolding. It is possible to get some pleasure from a chord sounding all on its own, but generally if you choose a favorite moment in a piece of music, and then omit everything that came before, playing only that one sound, the impact is diminished. A tune played with one finger on a piano can be enjoyable, though the individual notes have no appeal in isolation. Visual perception likewise can work on temporal structure alone. The Swedish psychologist Gunnar Johansson has made impressive films of black-clad people walking in the dark with small lights attached to their joints: shoulders, elbows, wrists, hips, knees, and ankles. As long as the person holds a static pose, we see nothing but a meaningless constellation of light spots. As soon as they start walking, though, they are revealed, as we vividly sense the unseen, moving human body. As always, however, what matters to the brain isn't perception but sensorimotor transformation. The brain has to transform temporal patterns of sensory signals into appropriate temporal patterns of muscle activation. It does this by shaping its neural networks into temporal operators.

Temporal operators differ from non-temporal, or 'algebraic', ones in that they respond not just to the current value of their input, but to the pattern of input over time. A differentiator, for instance, is a temporal operator whose output is the rate of change of its input. To a differentiator the instantaneous input is irrelevant; all that matters is how fast that input is rising or falling. An example is a speedometer, which doesn't care about the current location of the car or the position of the wheels, but whose dial indicates how fast the wheels are turning. For other operators it is other aspects of temporal structure that matter. But algebraic operators sense only the input of the moment. An algebraic operator is doomed to deliver the same output every time it receives a given input: the square of 2 is always 4, the cosine of 0 is always 1. Only a temporal operator can respond differently to the same instantaneous input, depending on past history. By this criterion it is easy to prove that the human brain is a temporal operator: greet a friend with the words 'Hi, how was your weekend?' and then, after they have responded, give them that same input again and listen for whether the response is identical. In our brains, complex temporal operators detect and create endlessly subtle temporal patterns. How do we do it?

Dynamic components

Brain, sensors, and muscles together make up one gigantic temporal operator, but neuroscientists tend to analyze it into simpler components familiar from physics and engineering. One of the simplest of these is the integrator. This is a device that accumulates the values of its input over time, so that its output reflects a sort of running total of all past inputs. An example of an integrator is a car odometer, which counts up axle rotations and keeps a tally of kilometers covered. Integration and differentiation are inverse operators: the reading on the odometer is the integral of the speedometer's reading, and the speedometer's reading is the rate of change of the odometer's. Differentiation turns position into velocity; integration turns velocity into position.

Another example of an integrator, and one that will lead to other ideas, is a bathtub. We can regard the flow rate of the water from the tap or shower nozzle as the input variable and the volume of water in the tub as the output. By playing with the tap, we can demonstrate the defining features of an integrator. For example, if the input to an integrator is a positive number, then its output increases; that is, as long as the tap is open, the water level rises. If the input is zero, the integrator holds a constant level. And if the input is negative then the output decreases—if we could get the nozzle to suck water back out of the tub, the level would fall.

Now suppose we loosen the plug, letting the water leak out. The rate of leakage will depend on the pressure in the tub, which in turn depends on the volume of water. The rate of change of the water level equals the rate of inflow from the shower nozzle minus the rate of leakage down the drain. The whole contraption behaves like a temporal operator called a leaky integrator, or low-pass filter. A leaky integrator responds to inputs in a dragged out, sluggish way. If the unplugged, or imperfectly plugged, tub is empty when the water suddenly begins to pour in at a constant rate, then the level starts to rise. But as it does, water leaks faster and faster out of the hole, so the water level inside the tub rises more and more slowly. Ultimately the water may overflow the edges of the tub, but if the inflow is moderate and the drain is large enough, the leakage from the tub will eventually become so fast that it perfectly matches the inflow from the nozzle. The water reaches a constant level, which it will hold as long as the inflow stays constant. If the flow is suddenly shut off, the water level will fall, quickly at first but then ever slower as the water pressure inside the tub drains away. This is typical of a leaky integrator: given any sudden, sustained change in its input, it drifts gradually to a new equilibrium.

Leaky integrators are also called low-pass filters because they respond to, or 'pass on', low-frequency inputs and they ignore high-frequency inputs. High-frequency inputs are ones that fluctuate rapidly, so that the leaky integrator, with its sluggish responses, can't keep up. Suppose the input is fluctuating about the zero line. No sooner does a positive blip set the filter's output ponderously rising than the fluctuating input becomes negative, drawing it back down again. In the face of this jittering input, the filter's output signal never moves any appreciable distance away from zero. Like a fat old dog playing with a puppy, it does essentially nothing. But if the input is low-frequency, slowly rising and falling, then the low-pass filter oscillates with it, though always with a delay. In the body, muscles are examples of low-pass filters; if you abruptly change the innervation of a muscle, your limb or head or eye will drift gradually to a new equilibrium position.

A high-pass filter in a sense does the opposite: it responds to abrupt changes but ignores sustained ones. Given a sudden jump in its input it reacts strongly, but if the input holds constant at the new value, the filter gradually loses interest and its activity drains away to zero. Human brains incorporate a lot of high-pass filters. The startle response is one: you jump out of your chair, but then settle down and cease to respond to the new status quo. When you jump in a lake to go swimming, you feel unpleasantly cold at first, then settle down, because your temperature sense incorporates high-pass filters. When you drive into a pulp-processing town on a summer's day, approaching the factory and the foamy, industrial river, you roll up the windows against the smell. But if you are stranded there, after a while your brain adjusts to be like the natives', so you can breathe through your nose and even eat in the restaurants. High-pass filters ignore low-frequency inputs—you aren't startled by slow, regular processes—but they react to every blip in high-frequency signals.

Dynamic order

There is an infinite variety of possible temporal operators, but they fit into an ordered scheme. Apart from a few exotica that seldom come up, all temporal operators can be defined in terms of two basic ones, the inverse operations of differentiation and integration. We set a prime beside a variable to represent its rate of change, so that x' is the rate of change of x (its velocity), and x'' is the rate of change of the rate of change (its acceleration) and so on. Then, for instance, the defining equation for a differentiator says that the output, y, is the rate of change of the input, x; in symbols, $y = x'$.

The equation for an integrator says that the rate of change of its output equals its input; $y' = x$. For a linear low-pass filter, the rate of change of the output is the difference between some constant multiples of the input and the output itself, $y' = ax - by$. For a linear high-pass filter, the equation is $y' = ax' - by$. The possibilities are endless: $f' = af - bf^2$ is a temporal operator that describes the growth of a fish population in a lake without predators but with limited space and fish food. By examining these equations or simulating them on a computer you can work out the dynamic behavior they express, but there is no need for us to do that here. The point is simply that there is order to the world of temporal processes—they can be built up from two operators and basic arithmetic. This is the ordering studied by Newton and his many followers, but it is not the only possible one. Later in this chapter I will argue that for computer-based neuroscience it may often be more convenient to use a different scheme, where dynamic operators are expressed not in terms of differentiators and integrators but of another elementary operator, namely delay.

Robinson's integrator

At his retirement party in 1993 D.A. Robinson, the Oculomotor Pope, was given, and forced to wear, a baseball cap bearing the mathematical symbol for an integrator. The cap commemorated Robinson's greatest discovery, the oculomotor integrator, which is a temporal operator built out of a looping network of neurons, whose existence he predicted on theoretical grounds in the late 1960s. He managed to locate parts of it in the brainstem fifteen years later. The first clues to its existence were found in the VOR.

VOR dynamics

As I said in Chapter 5, the VOR counterrotates the eyeballs when the head turns so as to keep the retinal images as stable as possible. The eye motion is driven by signals from the semicircular canals in the inner ear, coding head velocity. The VOR's job is to make eye velocity equal -1 times the head velocity, so that the gaze line remains stationary relative to the surroundings.[78] In the special case where the head velocity is zero, the eye must of course hold still in the head. So if the head turns and then stops, the brain has to counterrotate the eye and then hold it steady in its final position in the socket. To hold the eye steady in an eccentric position, the brain has to send a command to the eye muscles to combat the elastic forces that pull the eye back toward straight ahead (you can sense for yourself that holding your eyes far eccentric is tiring work). The neural command must be precisely matched to the position of the eye. But where does the eye-position command come from, given that the drive to the VOR comes from the semicircular canals, which carry information about head velocity, not eye position?

Robinson realized that the brain computes an eye-position command from the canal's head-velocity signal. It multiplies head velocity by -1 to provide an eye-velocity command, and sends the eye-velocity command through an integrator. Integration, remember, is the process that turns velocity into position, so the output is a continuously updated eye-position signal. Like a neural odometer, the integrator takes in eye-velocity signals and keeps a running track of the changing position of the eye. Given the neural integrator, the pieces of the VOR lock together properly: eye-position and eye-velocity signals together drive the motor neurons and muscles, and the result is an optimized reflex that counters the head's motion when it is moving and holds the eye still when the head stops.

Robinson and others sought the integrator's location. Single-cell recordings revealed neurons in the brainstem that receive eye-velocity signals as input and carry, in their own firing rates, information about eye position.[79-81] Damage to these regions causes the deficits you would expect after integrator damage: subjects have an abnormal VOR and can't hold eccentric eye positions—a syndrome called gaze-paretic nystagmus.[81-83] The same deficits turn up after cerebellar damage, suggesting that the integrator isn't confined to any one nucleus but involves several centers joined by loops.[84]

Velocity storage

Another temporal operator in the brain is called velocity storage. If someone spins you in the dark, in a rotary chair, at a constant speed, your sense of self-motion lasts for only about 40 seconds. After that it seems to you that you have come to a halt. Your VOR is also fooled: it stops counterrotating your eyes. The reason is that the semicircular canals are not perfect transducers of head velocity. Instead, they are high-pass filters: given a constant-velocity input, canal activity is strong at first but then dies away. Funny thing is, canal activity dies away in only about 20 seconds, yet your VOR and your sense of rotation persist twice as long.[85] What is driving the perception and the eye movement if your canals are silent? No other sensors are involved. Rather, the mechanism is a simple form of memory, a recollection of bygone sensor activity preserved in a reverberating brain circuit called velocity storage. Velocity storage is another temporal operator, in fact another neural integrator or low-pass filter, possibly built from loops that connect the vestibular nuclei on the two sides of the brain. Its purpose is to cancel, in part, the high-pass filtering performed by the sensors.

Optokinesis

Even with velocity storage the VOR is still too much of a high-pass filter to cope with sustained head rotation. But its errors are corrected by a low-pass visual reflex called optokinesis, which accelerates the eyes to annul retinal slip.

Optokinesis monitors patterns of image flow on the retina, and its visual processors try to deduce the head motion that might have caused that flow. This is a difficult job, and the processors can be fooled, as is evident in a striking illusion reported by Baingo Pinna and Gavin Brelstaff.[86] If you look at the central dot in Fig. 6.1 and move your face toward or away from the paper, you will see illusory rotations in the encircling rings.

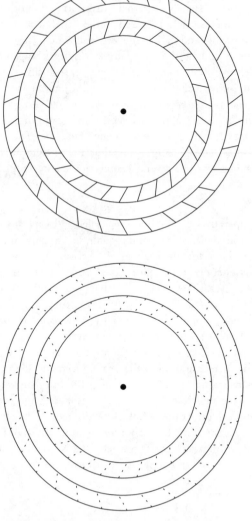

Fig. 6.1 Pinna and Brelstaff's illusion. Look at the upper dot and move your face toward and away from the paper; the encircling rings will seem to turn. With the lower dot the effect is weaker because the broken lines provide less-ambiguous local features.

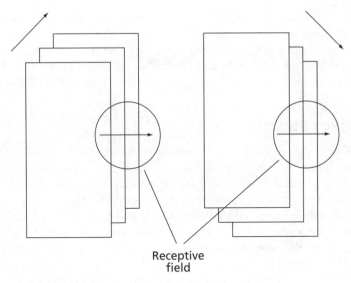

Receptive
field

Fig. 6.2 The aperture problem.

The illusion likely arises because each motion processor sees only a small patch of retina, or it assigns velocities to small features of the image, whose motions can be ambiguous. For instance, suppose a processor sees a segment of a moving edge but not its end points. Then there is no way to determine the direction in which the edge is moving, as you can see in Fig. 6.2 where different motions cause identical visual stimuli within the processor's receptive field. This is called the aperture problem.[87] Our visual system tends to assume that the motion is orthogonal to local lines, edges or other image elements. So in Fig. 6.1, the oblique spokes fool it into diagnosing rotary motion.

Even if the visual processors correctly piece together the pattern of image flow they may still confuse self-motion and motion of the surroundings. If you sit stationary inside a turning drum, watching its walls revolving around you, you soon come to feel that it is you, not the drum, that is rotating. This illusion, called vection, is the same one that makes you think you are moving when you watch IMAX films or when you see the train next to yours start to pull out of the station. Whenever a large part of your visual field moves *en bloc* your brain interprets it as self-motion, because normally that is the right interpretation. In the natural world, your visual field hardly ever moves *en bloc* unless you yourself are moving. The rare exceptions—staring down into a river or up at drifting clouds—cause illusions of self-motion.

Normally, though, optokinesis provides a useful visual backup to the VOR, accelerating the eyes when the vestibular reflex fails to eliminate retinal slip. Optokinesis is too slow to handle gaze stabilization all by itself, but it is useful for dealing with sustained head motion, when the temporal filtering in the semicircular canals makes the VOR unreliable. So the two gaze-stabilizing systems are temporally complementary: the VOR handles high-frequency motion and optokinesis deals with the low frequencies.[88]

Dynamic networks

How can the brain build integrators and other temporal operators out of neurons? There are two ways. It can use individual neurons that have the temporal properties it needs. Or, if its neurons can't do what it wants all by themselves, it can link them together in loops. With loops, it is possible to build temporal operators even out of purely algebraic (that is, non-temporal) neurons. Activity reverberates around the loops, creating a sort of memory of past inputs, so the network's outputs depend not only on the instantaneous value of its inputs but also on their past values. Both mechanisms—dynamic neurons and loops—are used in the brain, but the loops are probably more important because they are so versatile: you can build almost any temporal operator you want by linking up cells in appropriate loops. The brain is full of loops, and one reason for this is that they allow flexible and versatile temporal operations.

Any temporal transformation that can be achieved by a network of dynamic neurons can also be approximated arbitrarily well by a network of algebraic neurons, suitably wired together. In that case, the dynamics all arise from the conduction delays between the neurons. Earlier I mentioned that you can build practically any temporal operator you want out of some combination of differentiators and integrators, but there is nothing very special about these operators. You can equally well take delays as your fundamental temporal operators and build any other operator you want out of some combination of them. We will see in a moment how this can work. In what follows, I will describe how to build temporal operators out of loops of algebraic neurons, just to show in principle how loops generate dynamics. The same principles hold in the brain, except that there the temporal properties depend on the intrinsic dynamics of the cells as well as on the loops.

Simulating time

Simulated in a digital computer, time ticks along in discrete steps, like the second-hand of most watches. But real time is smooth, or at least extremely fine-grained. To make our digital simulations better reflect temporal smoothness, we can use a small time scale, letting each tick represent a millisecond, or a microsecond, nanosecond, picosecond, or whatever. But the smaller the steps, the longer our simulations take to run. If each tick represents a picosecond, our program takes a million million steps to depict 1 s of real time. Often the wait isn't worth it: round-off error in the million million computations builds up so high that our simulations lose all contact with reality. Sophisticated algorithms have been designed for the digital simulation of smooth temporal flow, but these are computationally expensive.[54] They slow down our simulations, and in the end they still approximate smoothness only imperfectly.

For most purposes in neuroscience I think we can dispense with smoothing and just pretend that time ticks along in discrete steps. Most of the temporal operators in neuroscience aren't known to any great precision, so it is a waste of time using fancy techniques to approximate an exact solution to a smooth equation that isn't accurate anyway. All we can hope is to simulate things well enough to discover the principles at work, and that, fortunately, isn't hard to do. In brain simulations, a slow, elaborate smoothing algorithm is seldom as useful as a simple time loop that can be programmed from scratch in a few key strokes and runs significantly faster. When I discuss temporal simulations, I will assume that time moves in discrete steps.

Integrating with loops

How can we build an integrator out of algebraic neurons? Calculus books contain formulae for integrating a few special functions, such as polynomials, sine, cosine, and so on. But our neural integrator has to be able to handle any pattern of input that comes its way, not just a few special functions, so none of these formulae are helpful. We need a general method, which we will get by returning to the definition of an integrator.

An integrator is what turns velocity to position. To convert an arbitrary velocity signal into position, you sample the velocity at close time intervals. Strictly speaking, the time steps should be infinitesimal, but for a brain simulation in a computer, a small interval, say a thousandth of a second, will suffice. You take a velocity reading and assume that it represents the average velocity since the last sample, 0.001s ago. As the step time is so small, you can safely assume that the velocity signal hasn't changed much and so this approximation is probably sound (if you are worried that your velocity signal does fluctuate on this time scale, choose a smaller interval). You multiply this velocity by the interval, 0.001s, to give the distance traveled in that time. To this distance you add a stored variable representing the total displacement since time zero. So the rule is, at each tick of the clock add the new velocity reading, times 0.001s, to the old displacement signal from 0.001s ago. This way, the displacement is continually incremented.

How could this be done with neurons? Imagine a network of, say, 100 cells, each taking its input from the same set of 1000 axons, whose collective firing codes a velocity. The network multiplies its input by 0.001 (that is, the synapses transmitting the velocity signal have that amplification factor, so each cell responds to 1000 input spikes with 1 output spike). To make the network into an integrator, we give it feedback loops: we make its axons loop around and synapse with its cell bodies, and we make the delay round the loops, from the input end of each neuron, out along its axon, and back to the input synapse, equal 0.001s. Finally we stipulate that the network's output—its firing rate—is the sum of the feedback and the multiplied velocity signal. So at any moment, its new output is its old output, from 0.001s ago, plus the velocity times 0.001—the same relation we devised for the integrator in the last paragraph. With this arrangement the network's output is, to a good approximation, the integral of its input.

For example, suppose the network's initial output is 0 and its input is constant at 10 000 spikes s^{-1} per cell, or 1 000 000 spikes s^{-1} for the network as a whole. At the next time step, 0.001s later, the network's output will be its old output plus the input times 0.001, which is 0 plus 1000, or 1000 spikes s^{-1}. After another time step, the output will be 2000 spikes s^{-1}. After a third time step, 3000. You see the pattern: given a constant positive input, the activity rises steadily, just as you would expect of an integrating network. Obviously if the input were negative the output would fall, and if the input were zero the output would hold for ever. These are the hallmarks of an integrator. The arrangement we used to build it, where the cells loop round and excite themselves, is called positive feedback.

Between leaks and explosions

The feedback loops make this network an integrator, but if the synapses on the feedback paths become too strong, even by a little, things go drastically awry. I assumed that the network excites itself with an amplification factor of 1; that is, when it receives no velocity signal its new output at every time step equals its old input, so it maintains a constant level of activity. If the amplification factor of the feedback synapses becomes even slightly greater than 1, the network's activity no longer holds a constant level but runs away to infinity. Suppose that the network's velocity input is 0 and its output is holding steady at 2000 spikes per second when the amplification factor suddenly rises to 1.1. At the next time step, the network's activity rises to 1.1 times the previous output, or 2200 spikes s^{-1}. Next round, it is 2420, then 2662, then 2928, mounting faster and faster at each step. Thanks to the miracle of exponential growth, after just 100 time steps (each lasting a ms) the individual cells' firing rates would exceed 27 000 spikes s^{-1}, if they could fire that hard. A network like this is unstable. Any positive input, however small and brief, can set in motion explosive growth, driving the output to its maximum level. This is a well-known problem with positive-feedback loops, as for example when the sound from an audio amplifier, picked up by a microphone and fed back through the amplifier, builds rapidly to a shattering screech. In other contexts explosive growth can have its uses, but in neural networks runaway firing rates are usually unwanted.

If the amplification in the feedback path falls below 1 we see the opposite pattern. In the absence of velocity input, the network's activity drains away to zero. Suppose that the network's velocity input is 0 and its output is holding steady at 2000 spikes s^{-1} when the amplification factor suddenly drops to 0.9. At the next time step, the network's activity falls to 1800 spikes s^{-1}, then 1620, then 1458, then 1312. After 100 time steps, the firing rate has dropped to 0.05 spikes s^{-1}. In the absence of input, then, its activity drains away to 0, though at a slower and slower rate. If the velocity input suddenly steps up to some constant, positive value, the network's activity will rise, fairly quickly at first but then more and more slowly, settling to a new equilibrium. This is the familiar pattern of a leaky integrator, or low-pass filter. In other words, we have managed to build a temporal filter from self-exciting neurons.

Building a perfect integrator is impossible in practice because the amplification can't be fixed precisely at 1. If it falls below 1, even slightly, we no longer have a perfect integrator but a low-pass filter. If it rises above 1, we have an unstable monster that runs away to infinity at the slightest nudge. The network balances on a knife edge between leaks and explosions. As leaks are the lesser evil, it is no surprise that Robinson's integrator and other known integrators in the brain turn out to be leaky. Deprived of input, Robinson's integrator loses its activity over about a minute. So if you try to hold an eccentric eye position in the dark, your eyes will drift toward straight ahead. To verify this for the Robinson integrator in your own brain, look at an eccentric object, or person, then close your eyes for a while and hold your head still. After 20 or 30 seconds, when you reopen your eyes, they will no longer be pointing at the object but will have drifted centrally. The demonstration doesn't always work, though; your eyes may drift centrally, but even in darkness that motion is detected by the brain, which may redirect the eyes back towards the unseen target.

Realism

Several authors, most notably Steve Cannon and D. A. Robinson, have simulated more realistic neural integrators.[89, 90] They recreate the firing patterns of real brainstem neurons; they approximate the intrinsic dynamics of the individual cells, treating them as linear low-pass filters; they use inhibitory rather than excitatory synapses, though the integration is still based on the same principle of positive feedback: pairs of neurons inhibit each other, so by inhibiting its own inhibitor, each cell is actually exciting itself.

Their models have helped us better understand neural integration, but even Cannon and Robinson's networks are still far from realistic. The real network in the brain contains far more complex, nonlinear neurons. The real network isn't even precisely an integrator, but some other operator, as yet imperfectly specified and certainly nonlinear. Deducing the behavior of

Cannon and Robinson's networks requires powerful mathematics, but these methods work only because the cells in the network, unrealistically, are linear. A truly realistic, nonlinear network wouldn't yield to the same tools. The real neural integrator is another example of an inscrutable network, best approached, I would suggest, by the techniques I have been advocating: identify the optimization principles and the error signal that shape the network, and then, if you are very ambitious, use computer simulations to help you explore its microscopic organization.

Learning dynamics

We know that the brain's temporal operators are adaptable. David Zee and colleagues rotated people horizontally back and forth inside a drum that was illuminated and patterned on the inside, so the subjects had something to see. The drum was itself programmed to rotate slightly out of phase with the subject's chair.[91] So the person in the drum saw an ebbing and flowing pattern of rotation which simulated more or less what they would see if their Robinson integrators malfunctioned, specifically if their integrators were abnormally leaky. I have experienced stimuli much like these, and I can attest to their ability to alter the viewer's brain: at first the flow pattern is mildly hypnotic, later nauseating, and it leads to a violent nystagmus in people whose eye control was perfectly normal half an hour earlier, before they sat in the fateful drum. What happens is that the brain, fooled into thinking that its integrator is leaking, tries to patch the non-existent leak. Its procedure isn't known for certain, but here is one option. I have said that a possible cause of integrator leaks in normal life is that the amplification factor in the feedback path drops too far below 1. Maybe the brain, fooled by the drum, decides that this amplification factor is too low, and raises it. (Of course in the brain the feedback loop doesn't contain 100 identical synapses, as in my illustration, but perhaps millions of diverse synapses, many of them possibly inhibitory, but the principle is the same.) Because the amplification factor was actually just fine, very slightly below 1, raising it brings us into the danger zone above 1. You would expect the integrator to become unstable, and this is what happens. People who have had this treatment can't hold a steady eye position to the left or right of straight ahead because their eyes are driven further eccentrically by their unstable integrators. When they try to look a little left, their gaze glides helplessly further and further left, and when they try to look a little right, it glides further and further right, until it hits the stops or until a quick movement—a saccade—resets the eye toward center. It takes time, exposure to the stable visual world, and a little lie-down to quell the nausea and recalibrate the integrator.

Velocity storage is also adaptable. This is probably the reason why it is weakened in figure skaters: when you spin them in the dark, their impression of motion lasts a shorter time than the 40s or thereabouts felt by the rest of us.[92, 93] In a way this is surprising, because velocity storage is meant to improve our vestibular sense, prolonging our impression of motion so that it better reflects our actual movements. You might think that skaters would need especially good motion sense, and should therefore have abnormally long velocity storage. But maybe the violent spins and sudden stops of figure skating are so far outside normal experience that our brains have no hope of representing them faithfully, even with souped-up velocity storage. So they adapt in the opposite direction, suppressing it. That way, they erase as quickly as possible all memory of the dreadful spin, and skate away afterwards unperturbed.

Mechanisms

Dynamics raises new issues for learning algorithms. In network simulations, there are two approaches: either train the loops or don't. You can build into the network from the beginning a set of looping structures that perform a variety of temporal operations—integration, differentiation, various sorts of filtering, and so on—and then leave them untouched for ever after. Learning would then consist of linking up the prefabricated temporal operators in different ways, but leaving unaltered those synapses that lie within the feedback loops. The other approach is to train both the synapses joining the operators and the synapses within them. Training the synapses within the loops is logistically more complex, but brings greater flexibility.

There is a variety of backprop that can be used to adapt synapses within the loops, but this algorithm is highly elaborate, and is therefore much less plausible biologically even than ordinary backprop, which is already considered suspect by most neuroscientists. The search for new alternatives is even more pressing here than it was in the previous chapter, where we considered algorithms for learning algebraic transformations, and found all of the current options wanting.

Furthermore, when the brain builds temporal operators it would be useful if it could alter not just its synapses, as in backprop, but also its membrane dynamics and conduction delays along its axons and dendrites. If the brain is capable of adjustments like these, then its learning algorithm transcends current versions of backprop, though it could still work on the same principle of gradient descent that I discussed in Chapter 5.

As you might expect, an aspect of learning that becomes especially critical when training temporal operators is timing. Even when we train a purely algebraic operator, say a network that adds two simultaneous inputs, timing matters in the sense that the network has to know which error signal goes with which output. If it got muddled up and started comparing its current outputs with the desired output for the *previous* input, mayhem would ensue. This sort of synchronization is more delicate for operators where the input and output are continuously unfolding in time. Little is known about how it might work.[94]

Another adaptive principle that becomes less trivial for dynamic networks is that ideally the error signal should vanish as soon as the network parameters—such as the synaptic weights—reach their optimal values. Therefore, the error signal should depend not on what has happened in the past but only on the network's performance in the most recent time step. We want, in other words, a temporally local error signal. When training an integrator, for instance, a poor choice of error signal would be the obvious one: the difference between the network's output and the integral of its input since time zero. Given that error signal, even if the network at some point stumbled across a set of parameters that allowed it to integrate perfectly, there would still be a large error, accumulated over the long interval before it learned its job. This error signal would continue to drive the evolution of the network parameters, propelling them well past their optimal values. A better error signal would be the difference between the current input and the rate of change of the network's output, because then the error would fall to zero the instant the network began to integrate properly. Presumably it was the job of natural selection to equip the protobrain with suitable, temporally local error signals.

Even with a temporally *non*-local error signal, dynamic networks can often be trained using a mechanism called teacher forcing.[95] Here, the error signals not only drive synaptic change, they also step in and alter the on-line performance of the network, like a ballet teacher manually adjusting the limbs of a pupil at the bar. For example, if the VOR malfunctions, rotating the eyes too slowly, then there will be retinal-image slip. The brain of course uses that slip to guide VOR adaptation, but more than that, the optokinetic system also measures the slip and immediately accelerates the eyes to compensate. Optokinesis resets the firing rates of the relevant neurons, or at least of some of them, toward the values they should have had if the VOR had been doing its job properly. It is this correction that is like the ballet teacher repositioning the dancer's limbs. The adjustment may simplify the learning task, and if the brain can distinguish neural activity due to the VOR from that due to optokinesis, it has an error signal for the activity generated by the VOR. It doesn't have to derive that error by back-propagation from downstream layers. In this way optokinesis may act like a teacher for the VOR, shaping the system into its correct behavior in a way that speeds up learning.

VOR models

In the last chapter I described Marr and Albus's ideas about cerebellar learning, but the mechanisms they proposed can't reshape looping networks to form temporal operators. Thomas Anastasio has devised a looping network that learns, by backprop, to perform the temporal operations, including integration, required of a VOR, or at least of a one-dimensional VOR that responds to horizontal head rotations with horizontal eye rotations.[96]

D. B. Arnold and none other than D. A. Robinson have described an alternative network that learns the same task without back-propagation, by a mechanism that its authors suggest may be more biological.[97] Unfortunately, one aspect of the model is disappointing: the authors couldn't get the network to develop both parts of the VOR—the integrator and the direct path carrying velocity commands—without stepping in and manipulating the error signal. They had to send different errors to different cells: unaltered retinal-slip signals to some and a low-pass filtered version of the same signal to the others. This device of distributing different teaching signals to different cells is essentially what the backprop algorithm does automatically. In backprop, the alteration at any one synapse depends not only on the error signal and the input to that synapse but also on information propagated from all downstream synapses, so the teaching signal that drives learning is different at every synapse. But where backprop adjusts these signals based on what is going on in the sensors and muscles and elsewhere in the network, Arnold and Robinson choose the distribution beforehand and hope it works.

If Arnold and Robinson's network were called upon to learn some other temporal operation, to cope with some change in the dynamics of the sensors or muscles or other parts of the brain, then its error signals would have to be specially adjusted again. So we are dealing here not with a general learning algorithm for temporal operators, as we were in Anastasio's model, but with a specialized set-up for developing one standard kind of circuit—integrators plus direct paths. It is like a restaurant that serves one dish, take it or leave it. I prefer something closer to Anastasio's notion that the VOR and other brain networks are flexible dynamic operators with more general-purpose learning mechanisms. To me, the adaptive flexibility of the VOR and other systems makes this idea more plausible. But at present it is largely a mystery what learning algorithm might provide that flexibility.

Chapter 7

Brains and brawn

God said, 'Let there be light' and there was light, but God is a special case. If you want light, you can't just will it; you have to proceed indirectly, for example by moving your feet and hands to search for a light switch. Outside your own nervous system, the only things you can reliably influence by a direct act of will are your skeletal muscles. These 656 muscles[98] are the main output path between you and the rest of the world—they are the user interface of the universe. Every command issued by your brain must be shaped to act through this layer. Much of what goes on in the late stages of sensorimotor transformations, the stages just before the motor neuron, can be understood as the brain's attempt to make optimal use of its interface.

Sliding filaments

Muscles generate motion by contracting. Of the three kinds of muscle in the human body, smooth, cardiac, and skeletal, I will discuss mainly skeletal muscle, which moves the limbs, head, and eyes. René Descartes believed muscles caused motion by blowing up like balloons ('I think therefore I expand'), but later measurements showed that muscle volume is essentially constant. The current leading theory of muscle contraction is the sliding-filament hypothesis, which is based on a better understanding of muscle anatomy.[99, 100]

Muscles are made of elongated cells called muscle fibers, and each fiber is composed of many long tubes divided into cylindrical sections. Running lengthwise inside these sections are protein filaments. When the muscle is activated, thick filaments, anchored at the middle, longitudinally, of the cylinder, reach out tiny 'arms' to grasp other, thin filaments anchored at one or the other end. The tiny arms pivot, release, and grip again further along, so that the thick filament crawls along the thin one, like a millipede climbing a string or a tug-of-war team dragging a rope, pulling the end of the cylinder toward its middle. Millions of filaments pulling in unison can create a lot of force and visibly contract the whole muscle.

To set your filaments in motion, you have to activate the muscles. One modern way to do this is by electric shocks: as advertised on TV, you wear a sort of electrified cummerbund that repeatedly zaps your stomach muscles, so you can develop washboard abs while sitting in the drive-through at Burger King. Similar methods may make it possible for people to control muscles that are paralyzed because their connections with the brain have been severed. But the usual, old-fashioned method of muscle activation is chemical: motor neurons release molecules of acetyl-choline which attach to muscle fibers. Attachment can be blocked by several drugs, causing paralysis. One of these drugs is curare, a resin from a tropical plant which has been used by Amazonian hunters to make poison blow-darts and by surgeons to immobilize patients who might other-wise flinch or try to escape. Another blocker of acetylcholine, but one that paralyzes smooth rather than skeletal muscle, is called belladonna, from the Italian for 'beautiful woman', because Italian women used it in eye drops to paralyze the muscles of the iris, enlarging the pupils and making the user more attractive. Bellouomo™, a supposedly analogous product for men, is in my opinion nothing but a complete waste of money.

In the absence of interfering drugs, acetylcholine attaches to the muscle cell, where it triggers a biochemical chain reaction that eventually sets the filaments in motion. The process draws its energy from adenosine triphos-phate (ATP) molecules in the cells. Without ATP, the thick filaments can't release their grasp on the thin filaments. In death, their unbreakable grip causes rigor mortis.

Forces of nature

These filaments, and other molecules like elastin and collagen in the tendons and muscle sheaths, create the mechanical properties of the muscle.[100, 101] Muscle exerts elastic force like a spring or a rubber sheet, pulling, when stretched, back toward its rest length. The more a muscle is activated by its nerve, the more force it exerts at any given length, but still the force varies as the muscle is stretched. So muscle is like a deluxe spring with adjustable properties. To see for yourself the elastic component of muscle force, grip a pencil as tightly as you can in one closed fist. You will find that it is harder to slide the pencil out of your clutch if your wrist is extended back rather than flexed forward, because wrist extension stretches the muscles whose long tendons work the fingers. In fact with your wrist fully flexed you can't even form a fist. I have seen this fact presented as a self-defense tip—it is said to be easier to prise a weapon from an assailant's grip if you somehow manage to flex their wrist, but this sounds more like a tip for getting your head blown off.

Muscle is also viscous, like glue: it resists fast deformations more than slow ones, so the pull it generates in response to any neural command depends not only on muscle length but also on how quickly the length is changing. A muscle creates more tension when it is stretching and less when it is contracting, and the faster it contracts, the less tension it exerts. You instinctively exploit this relation to extract more force from your leg extensors whenever you jump. When you want to jump upward, you begin by bending your knees. The idea is partly to stretch your knee-extensor muscles—your quadriceps—so as to exploit their elasticity, and partly to give yourself time to exert force on the floor before your legs reach full extension. But the third factor is muscle velocity: even when you jump from a deep crouch, you start by bobbing even deeper so that your knee extensors will be lengthening when you activate them for the jump.[102]

So muscle is viscoelastic: a bit like a spring and bit like glue. A better analogy is a Stretch Armstrong doll. This is a children's action figure with a rubber skin and a syrupy interior; the skin is elastic and the syrup is viscous, so a Stretch Armstrong behaves like a real muscle, though it can't adjust its own elasticity and viscosity by an act of will because it has no sliding filaments and no nervous system. (If it did, and if Roger Penrose's mind were transferred into its brain, he could contribute to physics for years in this form, until his rubber skin burst, releasing the syrup.) What do these muscle properties mean for a being with a brain? That is a question of mechanics.

Aristotle, Newton, and Euler

In the 17th and 18th centuries, Isaac Newton and Leonhard Euler (pronounced 'Oiler') paved the way for modern sensorimotor science by working out the natural laws that govern force and motion. Refined by later physicists, their work developed into the theory now called classical mechanics. As an exact description of nature the theory has been superseded by relativistic and quantum mechanics, but for everyday jobs including motor control and, apparently, the engineering of the Apollo moon missions, classical mechanics is entirely adequate.

The fundamental equation is Newton's second law of motion, which says that force equals mass times acceleration.[103] So if a particular force accelerates a 1 kg mass at 10 m s^{-2}, the same force will accelerate a 2 kg mass at just 5 m s^{-2}. Newton's law implies that a body driven by a constant force undergoes constant acceleration. In particular, a body acted upon by no force undergoes no acceleration: it neither speeds up, slows down, nor changes direction. So if a starship is flying at a million kilometers per hour through empty space, outside any net force field, and the captain shuts off the engines, the speed and bearing will stay constant. The same doesn't hold for your car, because the force of friction from the road slows you down. This observation misled Aristotle, and many other drivers throughout history, into mistakenly believing that constant-velocity motion requires force input, and that force determines velocity. Aristotle must not have spent much time in a kayak, because a few minutes of unintentional

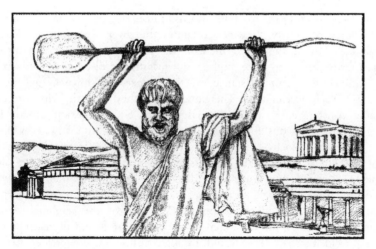

Fig. 7.1 Aristotle.

zig-zagging through the water shows you that your vigorous paddling isn't clearly reflected in your speed or direction but does have some faint influence on the rates of change of your speed and direction. On the other hand, maybe Aristotle *was* a master of the kayak, maybe he could do the 'Eskimo roll', but he failed to draw the right conclusions. We know he was aware of another, and to modern eyes clear, contradiction to his views of motion—he knew that an arrow continues to move long after it has lost contact with the bowstring—but he found the inspiration to explain this away: he said the string projected a beam of force onto the arrow that continued to propel it.

Driving force

The relation between brain activity and muscle action is complex and not fully understood, but a useful approach is to think of neural commands creating contractile force in the sliding filaments; this one neurally-controlled driving force then acts within a context of other forces, some arising from the muscles themselves and other tissues, some from outside the body. For instance muscle contraction always has to act against viscosity. As I have said, a viscous force is one that increases with the velocity of the object it affects; examples are friction and air resistance. In human motion, the main viscous forces come from the muscles and tendons themselves. If the joints are healthy, their articular surfaces are so smooth and lubricated that they are virtually frictionless.

If a second force, which I will call the *driving force*, is applied to a body subject to viscous resistance, then the driving force will determine not the body's acceleration but its velocity. A sky-diver dropping out of an airplane is subject to the viscous force of air resistance and the driving force of gravity. Gravity accelerates the diver according to Newton's second law, but as the speed increases so too does the retarding force of air resistance; the net force pulling downward decreases and the acceleration declines. Soon air resistance exactly balances the force of gravity, and the diver stops accelerating. Thereafter, until they pull the rip cord, they fall at a constant rate called terminal velocity. So, a constant driving force acting against a viscous force yields a brief acceleration followed by a constant, terminal velocity. For a sky-diver in free-fall, terminal velocity is about 200 km h^{-1}, though it depends on posture—a diver falls more slowly if they are spread out horizontally like a flying squirrel than if they are curled up in cannonball formation or extended like a vertical torpedo. Terminal velocity also depends on the viscosity of the medium. A diver dropped into a well full of water or a column of glue will reach a lower terminal velocity than they would in air, because of the greater viscosity. Conversely, increasing the driving force by encasing the diver in a heavy, lead suit or by amplifying the Earth's gravitational field will increase the terminal velocity.

So while Newton tells us that total force determines acceleration, we are often more concerned with the effects of a particular driving force, and in a viscous system the driving force determines not the acceleration but the terminal, or steady-state, velocity. Something similar holds for elastic forces. Imagine a bungee jumper hanging motionless at the end of their rubber cord. If you supplement the driving force by pulling down on the jumper's head, stretching the cord, then they will quickly come to equilibrium at the position where the elastic force of the cord exactly balances the new driving force. For an elastic system, then, driving force determines steady-state position. These principles are important for motor control, where the driving force of muscle contraction acts against the elasticity and viscosity of the muscles and tendons.

Speed and accuracy

To see what these principles mean for the brain, I will consider a simple motor task that is critical for survival. The task is to get some body part, say an eye or a limb, from position a to b as fast as possible without overshooting. We do this quite often with our limbs, and about three times per second with our eyes. I want to show that the optimal pattern of driving force for this task depends heavily on the mechanics of the apparatus being controlled. I will start with some simple cases, then move toward biological realism.

Consider first a purely elastic system, for instance a ping-pong ball on a spring on a smooth tabletop. Some particular driving force will hold the ball in position a, and another will hold it in position b. The optimal strategy for moving from a to b is just to change the driving force from level a to level b as fast as possible. The ball will snap from position a to b in synchrony with the force profile. So the optimal pattern of driving force is a step.

Fast and variable wins the race

Next consider a purely viscous system: a ping-pong ball floating submerged in a tank of glue. In this case the driving force determines the velocity of the ball. No force is required to hold the ball stationary in any position, a or b or anywhere else in the tank. Assuming there is some upper limit to the driving force we can generate, the optimal strategy is to exert the maximum force, driving the ball as quickly as possible until it arrives at position b, and then abruptly shut off the driving force completely. So in this case the optimal pattern of driving force is a pulse.

An inertial system is one whose responses are dominated by mass because other mechanical factors like elasticity and viscosity are negligible. An example is a heavy cart on a smooth, level road (Fig. 7.2). Now the optimal force profile is biphasic. You first exert maximum force in the forward direction, accelerating the cart as fast as possible. Then, halfway to b, you abruptly reverse the driving force, pulling as hard as you can in the backwards direction to brake the cart's motion and bring it to a halt at b. Remember that the task is to get the cart to b as quickly as possible and stop there without overshooting. If we didn't care about overshooting, we would just push all-out the whole way, accelerating the cart faster and faster. But if we want to stop at b, if we imagine that just beyond b is the edge of a cliff, then we need the biphasic profile: an onward pulse of force followed by a backward pulse.

So there is no room for half measures when you are trying to squeeze maximum speed out of a viscous or inertial system: during the movement you are always either pushing as hard as you can or pulling as hard as you can, slamming from one to the other instantly. This is called bang-bang control. To a good approximation, the same principle governs car racing, where the drivers are always more or less flooring the gas pedal or slamming on the brakes. It turns out that bang-bang control is always the fastest way to get a linear system from a to b, though for some nonlinear systems other control strategies may be better.

An enlightening variant is to push the cart up a slope from a to b as fast as possible without overshooting. For many people, their first instinct is that now we will have to push even harder during the acceleration phase, but of course we can't, because on level ground we were already exerting maximum force in keeping with the bang-bang principle. The other instinct is that we won't have to pull back quite so hard during the deceleration phase, because now gravity will help slow the cart. This instinct also is wrong. Of course gravity will help slow the cart, but if we find we can pull less than maximally and still bring the cart to a halt at

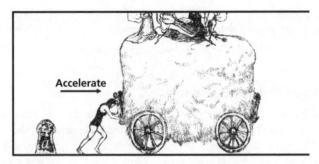

Fig. 7.2 The time-optimal force profile for an inertial system is biphasic: accelerate then brake.

b that means we could have prolonged the acceleration phase a little, and reached b even faster. The proper force profile is still bang-bang: push as hard as we can until the critical instant, now some time *after* the midpoint of the trip, and then pull back as hard as we can until the cart slams to a stop at b.

These examples show that the same quick step from a to b calls for entirely different force profiles—step, pulse, or biphasic—depending on the elasticity, viscosity, mass, and gravity involved.

The saccadic pulse-step

The simplest biological example of a fast, accurate movement from a to b is a saccade, which snaps the gaze line from one object to another. Saccades need to be fast, in part to get the eyes pointed at their new target as soon as possible and also because our eyes are like cameras with slow shutters. When the eye is moving between targets, our retinal images are so blurred that we can't see properly. So having made saccades fast, natural selection pressed for even greater speed, to abbreviate as much as possible the blind intervals during the motion.

In this case the mechanical system, the eyeball in its sling of muscles and connective tissue, is viscoelastic. Inertia plays no major role: because the eyeball weighs so little, almost all the muscle work goes to combat elasticity and viscosity.[104, 105] Mechanically, the eye is like a ping-pong ball attached to big springs and immersed in glue. Because the mass is so negligible compared with the elasticity and viscosity, even a special, weighted contact lens that increases the eyeball's inertia almost 100-fold scarcely affects its motion.

What is the optimal force profile to move this viscoelastic system as fast and accurately as possible from a to b? It is a mixture of the pure viscous

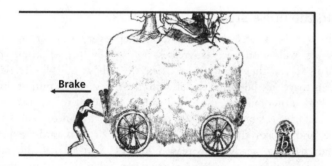

and elastic patterns we have just seen. The driving force starts at a level appropriate to balance the elastic force in position a, and it ends at a level appropriate for position b. *En route*, there is a maximal pulse of force to drive the system as quickly as possible against the viscosity. Actual force profiles during saccades, measured by strain gauges applied to the eye muscles of human volunteers undergoing surgery, show this pulse-step pattern.[106, 107]

The pulse-step pattern for saccades is seen not just in the activity of the eye muscles but also in the firing rates of the motor neurons.[108] During saccades, the motor neurons show a pulse of high-frequency firing. When that is over, at the end of the saccade, the neurons settle to a new, steady level of firing appropriate to the new eye position—this is the step. The pulse creates eye velocity; the step holds the new eye position.

These two components come from different sources. We have seen that during the VOR, the eye-velocity command comes to the motor neurons from cells in the vestibular nucleus. But during saccades, it comes from short-lead burst neurons in the pons and midbrain.[109] Burst cells are silent except during saccades in their on-directions, when they fire furiously at up to 1000 spikes s^{-1} in brief bursts that last as long as the saccade. These cells project to and excite the motor neurons that move the eye. They also project to Robinson's integrator, which converts their pulsed eye-velocity command into the eye-position command needed for the step.

So the brain uses Robinson's integrator to create the step component of motor-neuron firing from the burst neuron's pulse. It does this because it knows that the eye muscles, being viscoelastic, will convert a pulse-step of activation into a rapid, steplike motion of the eye. In every sensorimotor system, part of the brain's job is to complement the temporal properties of the sensors and effectors, fitting between them like a piece of a jigsaw puzzle, so that the overall transformation is optimized.

Learning the pulse-step

The brain creates a precisely tuned pulse-step every time it makes a saccade. As we will soon see, it creates an equally precise triple pulse of neural firing every time it wants to flex the elbow quickly. These temporal patterns have to be fitted exactly to their respective output interfaces, the eye and arm muscles, so they must be able to adapt when the interface changes. Damaging an eye muscle, for instance, makes saccades inaccurate and causes the eye to drift onward or backward after saccades rather than holding steady. The reason for the drift is that the pulse and step of neural firing are no longer correctly balanced to suit the altered mechanics of the interface. Pulse and step are now mismatched: the pulse drives the eye to a position that the step can't hold. Given several hours or days, the system adapts and the drift subsides. This ability to correct pulse-step mismatch is lost when there is damage to a part of the cerebellum called the flocculus.[64] Floccular damage often causes post-saccadic drift, presumably because the patient loses recent adjustments to the pulse-step generator.

How does the brain learn the optimal patterns of neural firing? The details are mostly unknown, but theoretically these patterns could be learned using simple error signals. Suitable signals could be based on motor error, which is the difference between the current position and the desired position, b. For some force systems, the integral of this difference would be an adequate error signal, because the way to minimize this integral is to get close to the target as fast as possible. With this error signal, an elastic system soon learns to generate the optimal step of driving force. Viscous and viscoelastic systems learn the correct pulses and pulse-steps. Systems that deal with a lot of inertia, like the arm controller, learn the wrong profile—they overshoot the target and then swing back—but they can be taught correctly by a slightly modified, and equally plausible, error signal: the integral of a nonlinear function of motor error. So time-optimal control can be learned from simple error signals.

The threefold pulse

I have written as though the pattern of muscular driving force faithfully reflected the commands issuing from the brain, but in fact the neural commands are distorted when they are transduced into force. Lloyd Partridge discovered that transduction acts like a low-pass filter: when the innervation steps suddenly to a new value, it takes a while, maybe a second or more in some cases, for the force to build to its new steady level.[110, 111] So really there are two layers of distortion between brain and world: transduction makes driving force a distorted reflection of brain activity, and mechanical factors like elasticity, viscosity, mass, and gravity make the body's motion a distorted reflection of driving force.[112] But the brain is aware of both layers, and has learned to work through them. The best example, I think, is the triple pulse of neural commands seen during quick arm movements.[113]

To flex your arm from position a to b, quickly and without overshooting, your brain sends a precisely timed triple pulse of activity to the biceps and triceps muscles, the flexor and extensor of the elbow. First it sends a burst of activation to biceps, then a second burst to triceps, and then a third to biceps again. Intuitively, the first two pulses seem easy to understand: number one gets your arm bending and number two brakes it. But what is the purpose of the third pulse? Some people call it a 'clamping' pulse,[114] but the word by itself isn't very helpful. Why do you have to clamp your arm? If you wanted to drive your car from a to b as fast possible without overshooting, would you first floor the gas pedal, then hit the brakes, then finally hit the gas again, to 'clamp' things? You shouldn't, because the optimal strategy is biphasic: accelerator then brake. So why does the brain move the arm with a triphasic command?

I think the key is the following pattern. We say that an inertial system is second-order, because the driving force determines acceleration, which is the second derivative of position, the range of change of the rate of change. More precisely, the system is second-order because the equation relating driving force to motion involves no derivative higher than the second. By the same criterion, a viscous system is first-order because its equation involves no derivative higher than the first, velocity. An elastic system is zeroth-order. We have seen that the time-optimal pattern of driving force is a double pulse for a second-order, inertial system, a single pulse for a first-order, viscous system, and zero pulses (but rather a step) for a zeroth-order, elastic system. So the pattern is that, for maximum speed, an nth-order system should be driven by a series of n pulses.

The arm, I suggest, is driven by a triple pulse because it is roughly a third-order system. Owing to its inertia, the equation relating arm motion to muscular driving force is second-order. And the transformation relating muscular driving force, in turn, to neural activity resembles a first-order low-pass filter. So the overall relation between arm motion and *innervation* is third-order, because it is a combination of the second- and first-order equations. For a third-order system of this type, time-optimal control requires a triple pulse.

We have little conscious insight into third-order systems, so it is hard to find everyday words, like the familiar second-order concepts *accelerate* and *brake*, that will help us understand what is going on. But with mathematics we can deduce the time-optimal drive for a third-order system. And the triple pulse we find in biceps and triceps suggests that the unconscious control mechanisms in the brain understand the situation perfectly.[114-116]

Torque

Most of our movements are composed of rotations at our joints, so what matters for motor control is not exactly muscle force but muscle torque, which is the rotary analog of force: torque is to rotation as force is to translational motion. Torque is produced by forces acting on bodies, though the same force, applied at different points on the body, generates different torques. If you nudge a ruler lying on your desk you get more torque for your effort, and therefore more rotation, if you push nearer the ends. That is why doorknobs are placed near the edges of doors away from the hinges. You also get more torque if you push at the correct angle. That is why you instinctively push into a door, or pull back, rather than yanking the knob up or down, or toward or away from the hinges, unless you are my Uncle Darren.

As you get more torque by pushing far from the hinge, you might expect muscles to capitalize on this principle by inserting far from the joints they rotate. By this reasoning the biceps muscle, which flexes the elbow, ought to insert close to the wrist. So why does it actually insert near the elbow? Maybe because natural selection hasn't managed to create muscles that are stretchy enough. If biceps ran from shoulder to wrist, it would have to shorten about sevenfold to bend the arm from full extension into full flexion, bringing the wrist up near the shoulder. Given its actual insertion, biceps can bend the arm that far with only a small change in its own length. And a fairly slow contraction of the muscle can swing the forearm at a high speed, like a baseball bat. So we are built in a way that lets small, slow muscle contractions generate big, fast movements. But the price we pay is an inefficient conversion of force into torque. Every time you bend your arm, it is like opening a door by pushing near the hinges.

Expert knowledge of rotary mechanics is built into the unconscious control systems in the brain, for instance the optokinetic system. If you are sitting motionless in a turning drum, experiencing the illusory self-rotation called vection, and the drum suddenly stops, then so does your vection and your optokinetic nystagmus. But if instead the lights go out while the drum is still turning, so that you have no visual information one way or the other about whether your illusory motion is still going on, your vection persists for up to half a minute, and you show afternystagmus: your eyes continue to track the invisible moving walls of the drum.[117, 118] In the absence of any visual information, your brain assumes that you are still spinning. The assumption makes perfect sense, because Euler's rotary version of Newton's first law says that a spinning body subject to no force will continue spinning with the same angular momentum. So when the lights go out, and your inner ear reports no braking force acting on the head, it is reasonable to assume that the (in this case illusory) rotation is continuing in the dark. Long before Newton's or Euler's discoveries, then, the law of the conservation of angular momentum was written into the sensorimotor circuits of the brain.

Meat head

I may be giving the impression that the muscles' main job is to make life difficult for the brain by distorting its commands, but really I expect that they provide something approaching an optimal interface, that they have been shaped by natural selection to ease the brain's computational burden as far as possible. When you reach for a jug of milk, for instance, and you underestimate its weight, your brain will program too little force. Your biceps will shorten less than you intended. But thanks to the intrinsic springiness of muscle, the stretched biceps will automatically deliver more force than it would have, had the motion gone according to plan, and this extra force should partially compensate for your brain's mistake.

There are probably many other instances, though it is hard to find clear examples given our current knowledge. One promising case involves Joel Miller and Joe Demer's finding that the muscles steering the eye run through connective tissue sheaths, or 'pulleys', attached to the bony wall of the eye socket.[119, 120] (Strictly speaking, these aren't proper pulleys at all. Pulleys are grooved wheels, but no one sees wheels in magnetic resonance images of the eye socket. More accurate names for Demer and Miller's discovery would be 'cringles' or 'grommets'.[121]) It has been suggested that the pulleys are carefully placed guide tubes which convert the eye muscles into a sort of mechanical computer which performs calculations that would otherwise fall to the brain. Several authors[119, 122-126] have pointed out ways in which muscle pulleys might influence eye control. It is still unclear which if any of these influences really explain the function of the pulleys, but it is a good bet that that function will turn out to be at least partly computational. And however the pulley story develops, the basic idea is sound that our musculature is designed to help the brain with its sensorimotor computations.

What sensorimotor computations could in principle be carried out by sets of muscles? Any computations at all. In theory, you could build a universal computer out of muscles, tendons, and bones. A friend of mine once built a computer out of toilet-paper rolls and paperclips. He says it worked well, though he now runs most of his applications on store-bought machines. In the 1980s a group at the Massachusetts Institute of Technology (MIT) made a computer out of Tinkertoys (a construction toy rather like Meccano)—I believe it is now their web server. In principle, entire sensorimotor transformations could be done mechanically. A whole brain could be built of muscles and bones, an intricate, levered contraption like a mad scientist's mousetrap. But natural selection avoided that path, probably because electrochemical computation with neurons is lighter, more compact, more energy efficient, faster, and more adaptable.

Learning through an interface

The existence of an output interface has repercussions for learning. Most efficient learning algorithms assume that the behavior that is being learned depends only on the network, and for most simulated networks this is true. But for the brain, the point of its activity is bodily motion, which depends not just on the brain but also on the muscular interface. How does this affect learning? In backprop learning, to take one example, information about the synapses in the output layer is propagated backward through the network. If the propagation were to miss the output layer and start a layer behind it in the interior, the algorithm would fail. So how can the brain learn anything, given that its final output layer is composed of muscle and bone? How can information about the transduction and mechanics of the interface be transmitted back to the adjustable synapses?

Actually the problem is much larger than this, because usually, the ultimate point of our brain activity is not even bodily motion itself but some consequence of the motion. In the case of your VOR, the point is to reduce retinal slip, and your success—your ability to drive down that error signal—depends not only on your brain and muscles but also on the optics of your eyes, on any glasses you may be wearing, and on the motion of your surroundings. Similarly, another error signal—perhaps some chemical disturbance in your blood—may trigger a chain of motor commands that is meant to find you food or a mate, and here your success will depend not only on your action but on many features of the wider world, including the distribution and behavior of potential nourishment or companions. In other words, the causal network connecting your sensory inputs to your error signals does not stop at your motor neurons or at your muscles or bones, but extends far out into your environment. How can learning algorithms work under these conditions?

The answer may be internal models. The brain could shape within itself a network that simulates the relation between neural activity and error signals. In the case of the VOR, the internal model might simulate the influence of the eye muscles, the rotating globe, any lenses or prisms before the eyes, and any foreseeable motions of the surroundings, in short everything it needs to predict retinal slip from neural activity. With an internal model like this, the brain would contain within itself a representation of the whole causal chain running from sensory inputs to error signals, and it could use this representation to run efficient learning algorithms like backprop and output-layer learning. If the internal model represented the processing performed by the muscles and everything thereafter, then the output layer of the brain, from the point of veiw of the learning algorithm, would be the motor neurons, because they are the final processing step before the muscles. But if the model represented also the processing in the motor neurons, then the brain's output layer, for the purposes of learning, would be the neurons one step upstream that project to the motor neurons. So interface models of this type would provide great flexibility regarding which cells in the brain could be considered output cells. Ideally, the internal model would be kept up to date when the real interface changed, so it would itself have to be adaptive, but this is feasible as the information needed to train the model—the error signal and all the neural activity from which that error is to be predicted—is available inside the brain.

Chapter 8

Thoughts running in circles

During the Second World War a mathematician named Norbert Wiener was recruited to lend his special talents to the American military effort. His secret mission: to design automatic aiming mechanisms for anti-aircraft guns. As he toiled over his sinister engines, with their sensors, motors, and electronic brains, he reflected that their operating principles applied equally to living organisms. After the war he presented his ideas in the influential book *Cybernetics: or Control and Communication in the Animal and the Machine*.[127] Wiener's central message in *Cybernetics* was the crucial role of feedback guidance, the process where a system's output loops back and affects its input to steer it to some goal. In this chapter I discuss why this sort of feedback is crucial to brain function. Then I broaden the perspective to show that feedback guidance is just one aspect of the larger concept of looping or iteration.

Feedback guidance

Typically a guidance system receives an input signal indicating the desired value of something, for instance the desired position of the eye (if you like, you can think of the word *desired* as an anthropomorphism, but a good case can be made that real human desires ultimately come down to signals driving feedback loops). And it has a part called a comparator which compares this desired value with the actual value of the same variable; the difference is processed further to compute the necessary adjustments.

In a domestic heating system the desired room temperature is set by the occupant turning a dial. The comparator is the thermostat, which compares desired with actual temperature, yielding an error signal. In this case the error is processed very simply: if the actual temperature is lower than the desired value then the boiler is switched on; if not, the boiler is switched off.

It is useful to consider an example where the variables are points in a two-dimensional plane, because interesting effects appear in two or more dimensions that don't come up in one dimension. For concreteness, we can think of our guidance system as a controller for two-dimensional (horizontal and vertical) eye position. The system generates an output, representing actual eye position, that is fed back and subtracted from the desired value, at the comparator, to give an error signal. To distinguish this signal that drives the motion of the eye from the error signals we talked about earlier that drive learning we will call it motor error (actually there is no deep distinction between the two, as learning is a special case of feedback guidance, but in learning it is usually synapses that are altered, whereas now I am considering guidance systems that directly alter neural firing rates). When the motor error is computed this way, by subtraction, the guidance system is said to work by negative feedback.

Guiding the eye

In preparation for later developments, Fig. 8.1 shows the motor-error signal from the comparator passing through an operator marked 'amplifier'. From the amplifier emerges a velocity command that rotates the eyeball. The idea is that the motor error, specifying the direction and distance of the desired position, or target, relative to the actual position, should determine the speed and direction of the eye. If the target is 10 degrees right of the eye's current position, then the motor error is 10 degrees right, and so the eye should move in a rightward direction. The velocity command is converted by an integrator into a position command. We know, from the last chapter, that there must be a positive feedback loop implementing the integration, so actually we have a positive feedback loop (not drawn here) nested inside a negative feedback loop, but for now we are interested in the outer loop. We assume that this feedback path has a strength of 1, meaning that the signal that reaches the comparator isn't magnified at all but equals the position command, or output, at the right side of the diagram.

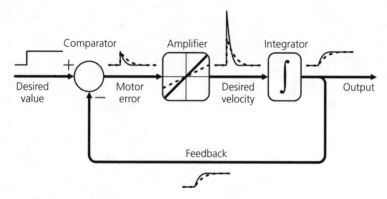

Fig. 8.1 A simple feedback-guidance system.

A computer simulation of this system is shown in Fig. 8.2A. At the center is an X-shaped target, and in the lower left corner a circle representing the eye. The system wants to drive the eye to the target. Fig. 8.2B shows the process in action, with eye position sampled at 1 ms intervals: the eye makes a beeline for its goal. Behind the scenes what happens is that the subtraction at the comparator yields a motor-error vector indicating that the target is up and to the right. The resulting velocity command drives the eye in this direction. At each succeeding time step, the eye is closer to the target, and so the motor error is getting smaller and smaller although its direction is unchanged. As the motor error shrinks, so does the velocity, with the result that the eye coasts in to the target ever more slowly. You can see this in the figure because the successive circles in the eye's trajectory, all sampled 1 ms apart, crowd closer and closer together. So a step in target position elicits a drawn-out, decelerating eye response. In fact, a feedback guidance system of this form is another example of a leaky integrator, or low-pass filter. We can speed up the motion by altering the amplifier that converts motor error into the eye-velocity command. If the amplification

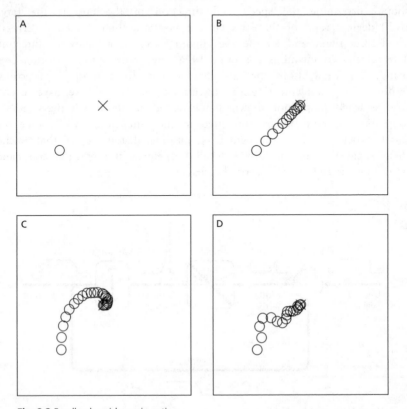

Fig. 8.2 Feedback guidance in action.

factor is doubled (see the solid traces in Fig. 8.1) the eye-velocity command for any given motor error will be twice as large as before, so the eye movement will proceed twice as fast, but still it will start quickly and then slow down in typical low-pass-filter fashion.

This decelerating response is not an invariable feature of feedback guidance. Guided missiles don't glide in like hummingbirds on their prey. To get a more uniform velocity out of the system, we can make the amplifier nonlinear so that it yields large outputs except for very small inputs. Now the velocity command remains large even when the motor error is shrinking. It decreases rather suddenly to zero only when the error becomes tiny. With this modification, the system no longer behaves like a low-pass filter, drifting lazily between equilibria, but instead snaps quickly into each new position. We will see that the brain uses this principle to speed saccades to their goals.

Internal malfunctions

Figure 8.2C illustrates what is probably the most interesting and useful property of feedback. In this simulation, the guidance system is seriously confused about the direction of the target. In the computer, I have simulated this confusion by rotating the motor error 45 degrees counterclockwise from the true direction of the target. In the brain, the cause might be signal corruption or malfunction in the pathways between the comparator and the integrator. You can see from the figure that the eye takes off at a 45 degree angle from the straight path but, steered by feedback, it curls in to the target. It curls in, even though the motor-error signals are off by 45 degrees throughout the movement. Obviously, a ballistic launcher that misaimed by 45 degrees would hit nowhere near the target (imagine a baseball pitcher with that sort of aim), but feedback guidance can work well even with very sloppy computation inside the loop.

What does this mean biologically? First, it means that feedback guidance can operate satisfactorily despite major lesions or malfunctions in its circuits. Second, feedback can guide a movement without perfect knowledge of the physical system being controlled. Even if your brain didn't know exactly what muscle activation patterns were appropriate to move your hand directly toward some object, it could send the limb in roughly the right direction and steer it visually to its goal. A third consequence is that feedback controllers can be built from simpler and faster components than ballistic systems (that is, systems without feedback guidance). There is no need for complex and time- or energy-consuming calculations of the precise launch direction. If you don't care about taking an efficient trajectory, all you need is a bargain-basement comparator that can find the error direction to within a 45 degree or even larger sector. With a larger inaccuracy, say 80 degrees, the eye would still reach the target, after a long spiraling trajectory. So there is wide room for error in a feedback-guided system.

But we shouldn't overestimate this error tolerance. For one thing, we may not want our eyes to spiral in gradually on their targets; we may want a faster route. Even if we weren't in a hurry, we couldn't tolerate inaccuracies much larger than 80 degrees. Near 90 degrees there is a critical angle that depends on various properties of the feedback system; if the comparator's inaccuracy is as large as this angle, the eye will circle the target eternally. If the inaccuracy gets any worse, the eye spirals outward to infinity. So fatal malfunctions are still possible inside a feedback loop. The lesson, I think, is that most neural guidance systems will still require fairly sophisticated processing within the loop. If visual feedback tells you that your hand is 5 cm right of its target, you still have to decide what to do about the problem—should you activate your brachioradialis muscle more or less, for instance? Decisions like these call for a lot of accurate information about arm geometry inside the feedback loop.

In short, feedback guidance probably permits somewhat simpler components within the feedback loop when everything is functioning normally, and it mitigates malfunctions in the case of injury.

Noise

Figure 8.2D shows what happens when the angle of deviation between the true and computed errors, fixed at 45 degrees in Fig. 8.2C, fluctuates randomly between 60 degrees clockwise and 60 degrees counterclockwise: it is a bumpy ride, but we get there. We can think of this random fluctuation as due to noise or unpredictable perturbations, so the behavior is analogous to a guided missile reaching its target despite buffeting winds. Noise is a bigger problem for limb movements than for eyes, because the limbs are more often jostled by varying and unpredictable loads, but even eye movements can be perturbed by noise within the brain itself.

Delay

The Achilles' heel of feedback guidance is delay. It takes time for information to get from the comparator to the output and then back to the comparator again via the feedback line. When this delay is too long—and how long is too long depends on many factors—then the comparator is steering the system based on outmoded information. The result can be overshoot and oscillation. You can see this principle at work in some showers where, when the water is a shade too hot, you can turn the cold tap astonishingly far with no apparent effect until suddenly you are standing in a jet of ice water. In feedback terminology, this is overshoot. A sensorimotor example comes up in the pursuit system, which rotates the eyes to track moving targets. It takes about 100 ms for visual information about a target to run from the retina through the various visual cortical areas to the extraocular motor neurons and eye muscles and produce an eye movement. This delay makes it impossible for pursuit to track targets oscillating at more than about one cycle per second. The quicker the movements, the more disastrous are the effects of delay, because news become obsolete sooner when you are moving fast. Long delays often rule out certain kinds of feedback in rapid tasks. For instance visual feedback is too slow to guide a baseball bat to a flying fastball.

Feedback in drawing

Our view of a process can change profoundly when we realize that it is under feedback control. Consider drawing. There is a story about one of the greatest of Renaissance painters, who was born Domenikos Theotokopoulos around 1541 in Fodele, Crete, but spent most of his working life in Spain, where he was known as El Greco. He is famous for his mostly religious pictures involving distinctive, elongated human characters. For centuries, people said that El Greco stretched his human figures to create a sense of heightened spirituality, or to correct for foreshortening when the pictures were hung high above the viewers' heads, all of which sounds entirely plausible. But in the 20th century a medical explanation was proposed for his style: it was suggested that he suffered from a deformity of the ocular lens which warped his retinal images. In other words, El Greco was simply painting what he saw.

This theory collapses when we realize that painting—or at least representational painting—is guided by feedback: the artist draws a line on the canvas and compares it visually with the model, or to memory or a mental image, making corrections if necessary. If El Greco's ocular lenses elongated his retinal images twofold, he might conceivably render a square window as a two-by-one rectangle, but then his painted rectangle would cast a four-by-one rectangular image on his retina. The artist, if he were aiming for geometric realism, would repaint it to make the retinal images of window and painting match. Even if his lenses had changed shape randomly from day to day, El Greco would still have been able to make accurate drawings from life. This fact is another instance of the ability of feedback systems to function in the presence of distortions and unpredictable perturbations.

Similar criticisms can be leveled against another popular art story, an early version of which is found in Giorgio Vasari's *Life of Giotto*, written in about 1568.[128] Giotto di Bondone was a fourteenth-century Florentine artist, one of the trailblazers of the Renaissance, famous even in his own time for his realism and his emphasis on the individuality, gesture, and facial expression of his characters. Vasari writes that a messenger from the Pope (Benedict XI, not D. A. Robinson) came to Giotto's workshop asking for a portfolio to take back to Rome. In reply, Giotto dipped his brush in red paint and 'with a twist of his hand drew such a perfect circle that it was a marvel to see.' The Pope, deeply impressed, summoned Giotto to Rome and 'recognized and honoured his genius'. A similar story is told of Pablo Picasso. The same theme of precise hand control turns up in Robertson Davies's novel *What's Bred in the Bone*, where the painter and forger Tancred Sarceni asks his new apprentice Francis Cornish to draw two crossing lines and then a third running exactly through the intersection.[129]

These stories are all based on the assumption that great artists must have great hand control. But do they? If drawing were a ballistic process, precise hand control would be crucial, but as drawing is actually feedback-guided, hand control beyond a certain minimum should be almost irrelevant. This again is the fundamental property of feedback systems, that accurate performance doesn't require accurate ballistic control. Studies of this question are few, but there is a 1956 film, called *Le Mystère Picasso*, that includes about an hour of the artist drawing on a special see-through screen where we can watch his picture take shape without his body blocking our view.[130] The film shows Picasso's fast, fluid, and, by the look of things, not very accurate lines racing over the drawing surface. When he retraces a line with a thicker brush, he misses the old contours very noticeably. His style is strikingly feedback-driven, and not at all ballistic: he constantly reworks and paints over. The whole performance supports the view that artistic skill resides less in the hand that draws than in the eye that judges whether the drawn line needs revision.

Opening the loop

Often it is possible to reveal the internal structure of a guidance system by artificially interrupting the feedback path, opening the loop. One example involves the optokinetic system, which rotates the eyes to track *en bloc* motion of large portions of the visual scene. As we saw in Chapter 6, when a large part of your visual world moves, which usually happens when your own body is in motion, your vision detects the speed and direction of retinal-image slip and accelerates or slows your eyes to reduce it. The causal loop makes this a feedback system: retinal slip influences the neural commands to the eye muscles, which then alter the eye velocity and therefore the retinal slip. In this feedback loop, the comparator is the retina, or more precisely the visual motion detectors a few synapses past the retina. Their output—a signal coding retinal-image slip—plays the role of motor error. So in this case motor error is the difference between desired eye velocity and actual eye velocity.

In the laboratory it is possible to interrupt the loop. One way is to immobilize one eye and block the other's vision with an eye patch. When the immobilized eye sees a moving pattern, the optokinetic system rotates the mobile but unseeing eye to try to track it. But of course the action is futile because that eye's motion has no effect on the retinal slip experienced by the stationary eye. The normal influence of eye motion on retinal slip is removed, breaking the feedback loop. When experiments like this are done on rabbits, even a small retinal slip leads to a steadily increasing eye velocity as the optokinetic system strives in vain to drive down the slip.[131] What does this behavior tell us? Any *algebraic* operator responds to a constant input with a constant output, so the fact that opto-kinetic eye velocity increases when the input, the retinal slip, is constant shows that the operator in the forward path of the optokinetic loop is dynamic, probably a leaky integrator. By opening the feedback path we can get at information about the operators within the loop.

An odd discovery regarding feedback guidance in drone flies involves a reflex of theirs that is akin to optokinesis.[132] Flies use optical flow to orient themselves. If they see the world streaming by to the right, they deduce that they themselves must be rotating left, so they move their legs and wings to turn themselves rightward. They accelerate rightward until their optical flow tells them they are again stationary relative to their surroundings. The scheme works well in normal fly life, but in 1949 Horst Mittelstaedt discovered that he could twist a fly's head 180 degrees on its thorax, turning it right upside down, and stick it there without killing or immobilizing the fly. Now the poor creature's optokinetic feedback drives it the wrong way. If the fly begins to turn slowly to the right, its upside-down eyes register what seems to them a rightward optical flow. The fly's brain deduces, incorrectly, that it is turning leftward. Apparently the fly doesn't correct for the odd posture of its head. Presumably it has never learned to do so because this posture is never adopted in normal life. To correct the illusory leftward rotation, the fly's legs and wings turn it faster to the right. Its optical flow increases further, causing the fly to turn still faster to the right. Soon the fly is spinning like a top, in a frantic dance, trying in vain to drive down its optokinetic motor error signals.[133] Needless to say, these flies make great pets.

Pursuit

Your brain has other feedback loops that you can open in the comfort of your living room. One of these loops drives pursuit eye movements, which, as we have seen, are the eye rotations we use to keep the images of small moving targets on our foveae, the high-acuity regions at the centers of our retinas. When you watch a bird fly, you are using pursuit. Only animals with foveae make pursuit movements. A rabbit, for example, doesn't have foveae, or at least not small round foveae like ours, and it won't track a small moving target with its eyes when its head is held stationary. But if the same rabbit is placed inside a rotating drum painted on the inside with stripes or spots so that the rabbit sees its entire visual field rotating *en bloc*, it will track the field rotation optokinetically. Humans have both pursuit and optokinesis, but pursuit dominates. When you track a small moving object against a detailed stationary background, say a rabbit running through the undergrowth, then optokinesis tries to lock your gaze on the stationary background, but it is overridden by pursuit.

Pursuit works well at speeds up to about 100 degrees per second. It responds slowly to unexpected changes: it takes about 100 ms to begin tracking a target that suddenly starts moving, which is why we need the faster-acting VOR to stabilize our eyes when our heads move. But the pursuit system can detect patterns of motion and use them to predict what is coming, so it quickly learns, while tracking a repetitively-moving target, to respond to changes in target velocity in much less than 100 ms, and even to anticipate changes.[134] Graham Barnes has shown how simple dynamic networks can achieve these predictions.[135]

Pursuit occupies a borderland between voluntary and involuntary action. Given a number of moving targets, you can choose to pursue any one you want, but in the absence of a target you can't normally will yourself to pursue. If you try to track an imaginary bird soaring across your visual field, you will make a series of jerky eye movements, saccades. So pursuit is like a reflex response to a moving object. Without a target, you can't pursue.

But the target needn't be visual. You can learn to pursue your own hand moving in darkness,[136-139] or targets that are cognitive rather than visual[136] (if you mount two lights on the rim of a black wheel and roll it across your visual field in darkness, you can pursue the hub of the wheel even though there is nothing to see there and even though neither of the two lights is ever moving with the same velocity as the hub).

Nor must the target be moving relative to the eye: if you stare very slightly to the left of a small bright light, say a light-bulb filament, for 10 seconds and then close your eyes, you will see a stationary afterimage, slightly off-center. If you try to look straight at the image, you will chase it to the right with pursuit. But of course the afterimage is fixed on your retina, and nothing your eye does can change its location. The normal connection between eye movement and retinal-image motion is broken, so your pursuit system is operating open-loop.

Feedback from the limbs

Limb movements are guided by feedback from sensors in the muscles and joints. Stretch receptors embedded in the muscle project to the spinal cord, activating the motor neurons to the stretched muscle and inhibiting the antagonist muscles. This is the stretch reflex, which physicians use to assess the motor circuitry in the spinal cord and brain. Tapping the tendon below your kneecap with a rubber hammer pulls on the quadriceps muscle, activating its stretch receptors. These excite motor neurons that quickly contract the muscle, extending the knee in a small kick. The exact role of the stretch reflex in normal motor control is controversial, but the logic of the knee jerk is clear: tendon stretch is detected by sensors; as the stretch was caused by a hammer and not by any neural command, it is at odds with the neural signals in the spinal cord coding desired limb position or muscle length, and so it evokes a corrective contraction of the stretched muscle.

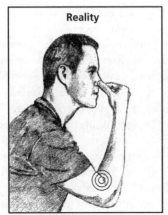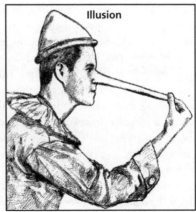

Fig. 8.3 The Pinocchio illusion: when your biceps tendon is stimulated your elbow feels more extended than it really is.

Feedback signals from the stretch receptors also enter consciousness and contribute to our sensations of body position. Abnormal stimulation of these sensors with a vibrator can lead to bizarre illusions.[140] If you hold a vibrator in the crook of your arm, it will excite stretch receptors in the biceps muscle, creating the impression that your elbow is further extended than it really is. One consequence is the Pinocchio illusion (Fig. 8.3): if you close your eyes and hold your nose while someone stimulates your biceps tendon in this way, you have the impression that your nose is ridiculously extended, because you can feel it between the fingers of your apparently extended arm. If you place a fingertip near your forehead while someone vibrates your triceps tendon on the back of your upper arm just above the elbow, you feel that your elbow is more flexed than it really is, and therefore that your fingertip is somewhere in the middle of your skull.

Internal feedback

Saccadic eye movements are too quick to be guided by visual feedback. They can be over in as little as two-hundredths of a second, whereas visual information takes much longer to make its way from the retina through the brain to the eye muscles. It follows that rapid gaze shifts can't be guided to their targets by vision. In fact we can make accurate saccades with no vision at all, to previously flashed targets in darkness. Nor are saccades guided by proprioception—our sense of our own eye position derived from sensors in our eye muscles. There are plenty of stretch receptors in the muscles whose signals the brain might have used to monitor eye position and guide saccades to their targets, but apparently it doesn't, maybe because proprioception is still too slow to guide the quickest saccades. In any case, complete loss of all proprioceptive signals from the eye muscles has little effect on saccades (at least immediately; it may be that proprioceptive signals contribute to adaptation).[141]

Saccades are believed to be under 'internal' feedback control.[108] According to this idea, put forward by D. A. Robinson, the eye-position commands emerging from the neural integrator are not only conveyed to the motor neurons and thence to the eye muscles, they are also fed back to provide upstream centers with information about eye position. That information is usually trustworthy because the eye, unlike the arm, doesn't carry different loads, so the same command from the integrator usually results in the same eye position. If there is a malfunction, if for instance the eye muscles are damaged, then the real eye position may not match the one commanded by the integrator, but if everything is working normally then the integrator provides an accurate estimate of the real position of the eye. Using motor commands in this way to provide feedback about the movement is called efference copy, because the information is carried by a copy of the motor, or efferent, command.

Efference copy plays a major role in perception. I have mentioned the vection illusion: when you go to an IMAX film and the whole visual scene rotates; you feel as though you are turning because your brain is fooled by the image flow. But when you use pursuit to track a rabbit against a backdrop of leaves and grass you don't feel as though you are moving, though the optical flow is much the same. Evidently the brain recognizes when optical flow arises from eye motion rather than whole-body motion. In the same way, when you look around a room or scan a page of print, it looks stable despite your rapidly changing retinal image, because the brain corrects for eye motion.

How do the visual motion processors know how fast and in what direction the eye is moving? Theoretically they could use proprioceptive signals from stretch sensors in the eye muscles, or they could use efference copy. Helmholtz argued for efference copy, based on this observation: if you close one eye, place a finger lightly against the lid of the other and gently jiggle the eyeball, the world does seem to jump around. So while the brain corrects for eye movements that you order through the usual neural channels, it fails to correct for eye movements where the normal efference-copy signals are absent.

In Robinson's model of the saccadic system, drawn in Fig. 8.4, the efference-copy signal from the integrator, coding the estimate of eye position, is fed back to a neural comparator. There it is subtracted from a signal, descending from higher centers, coding the desired position of the eye. The resulting error signal, the motor error, drives the short-lead burst neurons. If the motor error is to the right, for example, those burst neurons are activated that drive the eye rightward. The saccade proceeds until the internal estimate of eye position, coded by the integrator, equals the desired position. At that moment the motor error becomes zero. Deprived of their input, the burst neurons fall silent and the eye stops moving. This type of feedback is

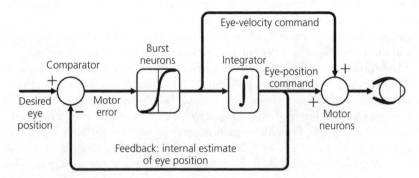

Fig. 8.4 Robinson's internal-feedback theory of the saccadic system.

called internal because the feedback signal coding the eye-position estimate comes not from any sensory receptors but from the motor circuits themselves.

Several pieces of evidence support this model. The firing rates of burst neurons correlate with motor error during saccades.[109] Brain diseases that damage the burst neurons cause not short, inaccurate saccades but long-duration, slow saccades that eventually reach their targets, as you would expect if the burst neurons were inside a feedback loop.[142] Silencing the burst neurons briefly in the middle of a saccade, by stimulating other cells that inhibit them, makes the saccade slow down or stop, but when the inhibition ceases the burst neurons come to life again and drive the saccade to near its target.[143] Stimulating horizontal burst cells briefly during a vertical saccade drives the eye off course, but when the stimulation ends the eye veers back toward its original target.[144]

Robinson's model has been extended and refined, most notably by Lance Optican, to reflect our expanding knowledge of brain activity.[145] The refinements will continue, because some things are still unclear. The source of the feedback signals is not known (there are possibilities besides the integrator). Nor is the location of the comparator; it may lie in the superior colliculus, in the cerebellum, or elsewhere, and there may be more than one. But the existence of internal feedback is pretty well established, and its functional advantage is clear: it allows feedback signals to reach the comparator quickly, because they don't have to pass through any sensors on their way; the loop is fast because it is entirely within the brain.

Iteration

The brain is built of loops, and loops within loops. Cells from central auditory and vestibular nuclei project back to the sensors that drive them, the hair cells in the inner ear. Axons from the visual cortex project back to the lateral geniculate nucleus. Wiring diagrams of the visual cortices show a welter of circuitry connecting many centers with one another bidirectionally. I have mentioned two reasons for this relentless looping: it allows the brain to have temporal operators and internal feedback. The third reason is that loops allow the brain to use a powerful computational principle called iteration.

Many problems in science and industry, and probably inside the brain as well, yield only to iterative algorithms. An example is equation solving, which comes up in every branch of science and technology. The simplest of all equations, probably first solved by the Sumerians, or maybe the Cro-Magnons, is the first-order equation $ax + b = 0$; the problem is to find the value of x for which $ax + b$ is 0. In this case, the solution is simple: $x = -b/a$. Next on the ladder of difficulty is the quadratic, or second-order, equation, which involves the second power of x, $ax^2 + bx + c = 0$. Now the solution is less obvious, but it was known to the Babylonians and it is familiar to most people nowadays as the quadratic formula from high-school math; the solution is $-b$ plus or minus the square root of $b^2 - 4ac$, all divided by $2a$. If the equation is cubic, or third-order, involving x to the third power, the solution becomes far more complex, but it is known; it was discovered in 1535 by the Italian mathematician and topographer Niccolò Tartaglia. For the fourth-order, or quartic, case, the solution was discovered in 1540 by Lodovico Ferrari. But after this burst of Italian algebra, progress came to a halt. Generations of mathematicians sought in vain the general solution to the fifth-order equation. Finally, in 1824, the Norwegian mathematician Niels Abel took another approach, and proved that there is in fact no solution. There simply is no formula for solving a fifth- or higher-order equation, no calculation based on the elementary operations of addition, subtraction, multiplication, division, and radicals (that is, computing square roots, cube roots, and so on).

Does this mean that all human technology, all our science and engineering, is for ever helpless in the face of equations beyond the fourth order? Not at all. Given an arbitrary fifth-order equation, say $x^5 + 3x^3 + 1 = 0$, I need only a moment on a computer, or a few minutes with pencil and paper, to compute by iteration that the root is -0.6625, to the fourth decimal place. The technique is quite different from the formulae devised by the Italians and the Greeks. Instead of a closed formula that yields an exact answer, it involves a series of guesses. We start with a guess and then improve it over and over by repeating a specific procedure. In this case the procedure is to consider the graph of the equation and compute the slope of the curve at some point x. We pretend that the curve is a straight line with that slope, and we step to a new point where that straight line crosses the x-axis; that is, we step to the root of that straight line. If the curve is not in fact a straight line, we won't land on the root we are seeking, but if we repeat this procedure over and over, it can bring us closer and closer to the root. For instance, given the above fifth-order equation, I might choose as my first guess the number $x = 1$. At this point, the height of the curve is $1^5 + 3 \times 1^3 + 1 = 5$. The slope of the curve here is easily computed; it is 14. A line of slope 14 running through this point would cross zero when x equals $1 - 5/14$, or 0.6429, so that becomes my new guess. Repeating the procedure, I generate the sequence, 1, 0.6429, 0.2259, −1.9655, −1.4983. −1.1317, −0.8679, −0.7167, −0.6673, −0.6626, −0.6625, −0.6625, −0.6625, and so on. By this method I can't calculate the root exactly, I can only approximate it, but as I can approximate to any level of precision I want that is usually good enough.

This pattern repeats throughout applied mathematics. Exact formulae work only in severely restricted cases, but problems of extreme generality can be handled using iterative, successive approximation. In the field of differential equations, linear cases and a few other special types can be solved by exact formulae, but all others need an iterative approach. Optimization is another example, where certain linear cases can be handled exactly by matrix inversion but almost all others call for an iterative algorithm such as gradient descent.

Why can iterative algorithms make headway when exact methods fail? For one thing, they are satisfied with approximate answers. For another, they decompose difficult problems into easier subproblems. In the case of optimization, for instance, finding the lowest point, or even a local optimum, in a complex energy landscape is a difficult problem, but gradient descent—simply finding the direction in which the surface is sloping down most quickly and taking a small step in that direction—is an easy problem. Solving the easy problem over and over again eventually brings us to a solution of the hard problem, finding an optimum.

One probable application of iterative algorithms in the brain is learning, as we saw in Chapter 5. In Chapter 11 I will mention another possible role for neural iteration, in piecing together a unified picture of the world from various sensory signals.

I have emphasized the power of iterative algorithms, but it is worth keeping in mind that no task, in itself, demands iteration. Whether iteration is needed depends on our repertoire of elementary operations such as addition, multiplication, and so on. A task that defies non-iterative solution in our addition and multiplication based mathematics might nevertheless be done without iteration given other basic operations. I have said that human mathematicians can solve fifth-order equations only iteratively, but if you owned a 'fifth-order equation solver', maybe culled from an alien spacecraft, then you wouldn't share that limitation. Similarly, just because a task calls for iteration in human mathematics doesn't necessarily mean that it is done iteratively in the brain.

But at the same time, whatever your array of elementary operations, even if you are working with a set of alien functions, still you will probably be able to increase your computational power by using iteration. The brain likely works with some finite set of basic operations; they aren't the same as our addition and multiplication, but whatever they are it is likely that iterative algorithms would greatly expand their capabilities. So it is not surprising that the brain is built for iteration.

Chapter 9

Degrees of freedom

In Edwin Abbott's *Flatland*,[146] an inhabitant of a two-dimensional world is bewildered by a visitor from the third dimension, a sphere intersecting his plane. He has never seen anything like it. To his two-dimensional mind, the very concept of a sphere makes no sense. In this chapter I will argue that we are like Flatlanders, studying multidimensional sensorimotor systems whose remarkable properties are invisible, in fact unthinkable, unless we look at them in all their degrees of freedom. Most sensorimotor research in the twentieth century restricted itself to one or two dimensions, for instance to horizontal or vertical eye motion, or to the angle of a single joint in a moving limb. Very sensibly, the researchers were simplifying a complex problem. But recent work has begun to lift us out of Flatland into a strange new sensorimotor world, though in many cases we are merely regaining earlier insights of nineteenth-century pioneers like Helmholtz, Fick, Donders, and Listing. I want to convey something of this strange new world, but my message is not going to be that all hell breaks loose in higher dimensions, that we can't hope to foresee the weirdness that unfolds whenever we consider a new degree of freedom. Instead I will argue that we can very well generalize from low to high dimensions if we generalize the right way, based on optimization.

Dimensions of mind

A thing has n dimensions, or degrees of freedom, if we need n numbers to describe it completely.[147] A moving particle has three degrees of freedom—if we are interested only in its location and not, say, its velocity or acceleration or mass or color—because a full description of the location requires three numbers: its coordinates along the three axes, north/south, east/west, and up/down. That is why we say physical space is three-dimensional.

Abstract spaces may have more than three dimensions. Until recently, it was said that humans sensed four basic flavors; so 'taste space' (not counting the contributions of smell to our experience of food) had four dimensions—sweet, sour, salty, and bitter. Now it seems that taste space is at least five-dimensional, with a newly discovered dimension called *umami*, or sometimes *meaty* or *delicious*.[148-150] It has likewise been suggested that our sense of smell works with a small set of basic categories—acrid, ethereal, floral, minty, musky, putrid, and resinous—making smell space seven-dimensional, but this categorization was never universally accepted, and newer research reveals genes, in mice and humans, for over 500 different olfactory receptor molecules, so our smell space may be higher-dimensional than we thought. In bright light, color space is at least three-dimensional, because the cones in our retinas contain three types of color-sensitive pigments, for red, green, and blue. In dim light our color space shrinks to one dimension, all gray, because only one type of photoreceptor, the rods, is active, and they contain just one light-sensitive pigment, called visual purple, so named because the chemical itself is purple though the visual sensations it evokes in our minds are gray. Some birds enjoy a four-dimensional color space. And so may some women, because they have two types of red receptors. Even for men, color space may have more than three dimensions. Iridescent colors may arise partly from rivalry, when the same spot on a surface sends different wavelengths to the two eyes; this binocular discrepancy is another dimension of information that expands our color space. In dreams, we see colors that were not evoked by activity in our rods and cones, so it is conceivable that unusual patterns in our visual cortices could then reveal exotic new dimensions of color space, but it is also possible that our central color circuitry is constrained, even in dreams, to deal in terms of the colors of waking life.

In physical space we need just three coordinates to specify the position of a single point, but our own bodies contain many points, so describing body position requires more than three numbers. How many more? A freely moving system comprising two points has six degrees of freedom, because we need three numbers to describe the location of each of the two points. A system of three points has nine degrees of freedom, and in general a collection of n points has $3n$ degrees of freedom. A human body has something like 7×10^{27} atoms. Even our heads hold 5×10^{26} atoms on average (mine has slightly more). Do we need 1.5×10^{27} numbers just to describe the position of the head? No, we can do better using constraints.

Constraints on freedom

Constraints are conditions which a system satisfies and which may reduce the number of its degrees of freedom. I said that two freely moving points have six degrees of freedom between them. Now suppose we have two particles which are not entirely free, but which obey the constraint that the distance between them is constant—imagine them joined by a rigid rod 1 m long. Because the points can't move toward or away from each other, they lose freedom. Three numbers specify the location of either one of the points. When that one point is fixed, the second is still free to move, but it is restricted to a sphere of radius 1 m, centered on the first point. To specify a point on a sphere we need two coordinates, for example longitude and latitude on the surface of the Earth, therefore the second point has two degrees of freedom once the location of the first point is determined. So five numbers are needed, in all, to describe the configuration of the two-point system. The constant-distance constraint has reduced the degrees of freedom of the two-point system from six to five.

Similar reasoning shows that a contraption of three points at fixed distances from one another, three particles joined in a triangle by three rigid rods, has six degrees of freedom. We have just seen that five numbers are needed to describe the positions of two of the three points. When those two points of the triangle are fixed, the third is severely restricted in its motion: it can only swing in a circle. A circle is one-dimensional, like a line, and so a single number suffices to indicate where the point is on it. In total, then, six numbers describe the configuration of the three-point system: three numbers for the first point, two for the second, and one for the third.

Remarkably, the number of degrees of freedom stays frozen at six no matter how many new points we introduce, as long as the points are constrained so that the distances between them don't change. A set of three or more points, in which the distances between all points are fixed, is called a rigid body. Many parts of the human body, for instance eyes, skull, and limb bones, are essentially rigid, except in wrestlers and stunt pilots, so their positions can be expressed with amazing efficiency, using just six numbers.

Moving in six dimensions

When I introduced the vestibulo-ocular reflex in Chapter 5, I said that rigid bodies undergo two kinds of motion: translation and rotation. Each of these motions has three degrees of freedom. This is why natural selection has designed us with three semicircular canals in each of our inner ears. Each canal measures one dimension of head rotation, so three canals are needed to report all three dimensions.

Why do we need two copies of these sensors, a set of three on each side of the head? That isn't quite so clear. The two sets complement each other: the horizontal canal on the right side can measure high speeds of rightward head spin, but its activity hits zero at low speeds of leftward spin, while the horizontal canal on the left side shows the opposite pattern, so between them the two canals cover a wider range of head velocity than either would alone—but that isn't much of an explanation, because presumably it would have been possible to evolve single canals with wider operating ranges. Another idea is that we have two sets of canals in case one set is damaged, just as we have two kidneys, two livers, two hearts . . . ; this explanation also is unsatisfying. More likely there are historical reasons for the arrangement. As I said earlier, the canals evolved out of something like the lateral line organ of fish, which very sensibly exists in two copies, on the two sides of the body, because the fish wants to sense ripples on both sides. (Why put the two sets of sensors on the two sides of the animal and not, say, front and back? Because the developmental machinery that builds the lateral line organ in the embryonic fish exploits an earlier adaptation that makes embryonic development roughly mirror symmetrical, with the mirror oriented in the animal's mid-sagittal plane.) On this view, the canal arrays are bilaterally symmetrical because they started out that way.

Oddly, though, it is possible to show that if you are committed to having mirror-symmetric sensor arrays on the two sides of your head, you could actually get by with just two canals on each side instead of three, for a total of four canals in all. The four-canal arrangement isn't intuitively obvious, but it is illustrated in Fig. 9.1. With a little study, you can verify that the four canals can encode any direction of head rotation. So why do we have six canals instead of four? Most likely for efficient coding. Given the same sensitivity and the same levels of noise, it can be shown that a set of sensory fibers innervating the four-canal array would need higher firing rates to convey the same information than they would if they innervated the six-canal array.

As for the otolith organs, there are two on each side of the head, a horizontal sheet of hair cells in the utricle and a vertical one in the saccule, each containing cells responsive to translation in various directions in

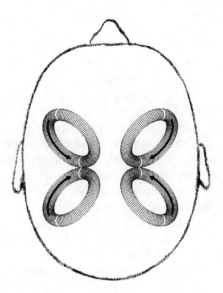

Fig. 9.1 Alternative-universe arrangement of vestibular sensors.

its particular plane. As each sheet senses two dimensions of head translation, the two sheets more than cover the three dimensions of translational motion that the head has in total. So the canals and otoliths together can handle all six dimensions of rotation and translation.

Translation and rotation are entirely different forms of motion. Even the fact that both have three degrees of freedom is a superficial similarity, a sort of accident that comes about because we happen to live in three-dimensional space. In two-dimensional space, translations have two degrees of freedom but rotations have just one: a flat, two-dimensional disk confined to a plane can rotate about only one axis, the one at right angles to the plane. In four-dimensional space, translations have four degrees of freedom but rotations have six. If we lived in a hyperspace of ten dimensions (as we may do, according to one of the less extravagant theories of modern physics) we would have no fewer than 45 degrees of freedom for rolling around.[151]

The twisting eye

Each eye has three degrees of freedom. It doesn't translate around your face but it rotates in three dimensions, horizontally, vertically, and sometimes torsionally, twisting about its own line of sight. If you roll your head clockwise (that is, right-ear down) then the VOR will twist your eyes counterclockwise in their sockets to keep your retinal image from rolling around its center. You can sometimes sense your own torsional eye rotations. Sit in a rotary office chair, lean your head back almost horizontally and look at the ceiling. If you now spin the chair with your feet, or have someone else do it, while you stare at a fixed point directly overhead, you may be able to sense the tiny jolts of your visual world every time your VOR resets your eye position with a torsional quick phase of nystagmus. You can do the demonstration without the chair by staring at a spot on the ceiling and slowly pirouetting beneath it.

You can also see your own twisting eye movements in a mirror. With your face up close to the glass, select one of the tiny blood vessels in the white of one eye. Roll your head slowly clockwise or counterclockwise, that is right- or left-ear down, and watch the vessel move relative to your eyelids as your eye counterrotates in its socket. The counterrotation is driven by two mechanisms. Your semicircular canals sense your head rotation and twist the eyes to compensate—this is the action of the VOR that we have discussed in earlier chapters. And your otolith organs sense the pull of gravity and twist your eyes toward upright when your head tilts—this is another aspect of the VOR, called the counterroll reflex. Counterroll is weak in humans.[152, 153] When you hold your head 90 degrees clockwise relative to gravity, for instance when you lie on your right side in bed, your eyes remain twisted only about 5 or 10 degrees counterclockwise. But the reflex may have been stronger in our evolutionary ancestors. It is still strong in rabbits, probably because their version of the fovea (the retinal region specialized for high-acuity vision) isn't small and round like ours but is elongated into a horizontal 'visual streak'. Rabbits use counterroll to keep their visual streaks roughly aligned with the horizon, so they can keep a look-out for predators approaching in the ground plane.

To achieve our three degrees of freedom, we use six muscles to steer each eye. Do we really need that many muscles? For some reason, the question is controversial. In his *Plan and Purpose in Nature*,[154] the great evolutionary theorist G. C. Williams presents the sextet of eye muscles as one of natural selection's gaffes. He says the eye could rotate just as well with only three muscles. No doubt Williams is right that natural selection sometimes lets us down, but presenting specific examples is always risky. The three-muscle plan that he and others favor is, I think, a tripod arrangement where the muscle insertions are spaced 120 degrees apart, forming an equilateral triangle when seen from in front. But this arrangement is inadequate because it can't twist the eye. All three of these muscles would rotate the eyeball about axes in the frontal plane; they would be unable to rotate it about its own line of sight. They would have no way to stabilize the retinal image when the head rolled sideways, and there would be other problems as well. A better option would be three muscles pulling at right angles to one another, say rightward, upward, and clockwise. But now the problem is that muscles can only pull, not push. If you wanted to snap your eye quickly to the left, the best you could do would be to relax your rightward-pulling muscle and let some arrangement of elastic ligaments on the other side of the eye pull it leftward. To achieve any reasonable leftward velocity, the ligaments would have to be very strong and stiff, which would mean that the rightward muscle would have to exert huge amounts of force to yank the eye right. Better to replace the ligaments by muscles whose forces can be controlled by the brain: make them pull hard to the left when you want to saccade left, relax when you want to saccade right. The result would be an arrangement of six muscle pairs, pulling right and left, up and down, clockwise and counterclockwise. This is what natural selection has provided us with, except that the whole arrangement is rotated about 45 degrees: our muscle pairs pull right and left, up-clockwise and down-counterclockwise, and up-counterclockwise and down-clockwise.[155]

Linkages

Not all our moving parts are rigid bodies. Our tongues are capable of flexing and curling movements which are outside the rigid-body repertoire. Our limbs also are pliant, but they are composed of chains, called linkages, of rigid bodies. The arm, for example, is made up of the bones humerus, radius, and ulna, and the many small bones in the hand.

Our skeletons are hooked together by five geometric types of mobile joint. Hinge joints permit rotation with one degree of freedom: the two connected links swing only about a single axis relative to one another.

Anatomical examples are the knee, the humero-ulnar joint of the elbow, and the two distal joints of each finger. Pivot joints also allow one degree of freedom but in this case one link rotates about its own long axis. An example is the radio-ulnar joint, where the radius (the forearm bone on the thumb side) turns in a tissue ring attached to the ulna. Saddle joints, like the one between the thumb and wrist, permit rotation with two degrees of freedom. Both articular surfaces are saddle-shaped: convex in one direction and concave in the other. Ellipsoidal joints like the wrist also allow two degrees of freedom. Their articular surfaces are ellipsoids, or elongated spheres. And ball-and-socket joints have three degrees of freedom. Examples are the eye in the orbit and the shoulder and hip joints.

Other types of joints are possible, but they don't occur in our bodies. Robots, for instance, can have prismatic joints, which slide like the segments of a collapsible telescope. But human joints are almost purely rotational. So if you ever stop for lunch in an unfamiliar small town and you notice that the townsfolk have prismatic joints, get out of there fast.

Any joint has an operating range beyond which it doesn't willingly move. For a hinge joint, you can specify the range by giving two angular limits; for instance the humero-ulnar joint allows angles between forearm and upper arm ranging from about 0 to 135 degrees. With this example I was introduced to biomechanics as a seven-year-old at Kingsway School, where a popular form of social interaction was for bigger students to extend smaller students' joints beyond their normal ranges.

In the absence of any extra constraints, the total number of degrees of freedom of a linkage is the sum of the degrees of freedom of its joints. Consider the arm. The shoulder has three degrees of freedom, because you can rotate your upper arm about three orthogonal axes: you can rotate it about a forward–backward axis, as when making snow angels; you can rotate it about the long axis of the body, as when doing push-ups; and you can twist your arms about their own long axes, as when you reach out

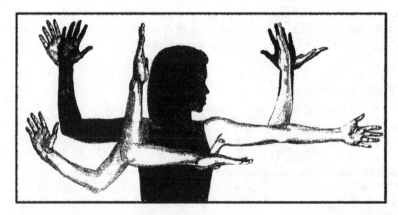

Fig. 9.2 The arm's seven degrees of freedom.

sideways and turn a doorknob, or when you sweep your arm like a windshield wiper before your face. The elbow has two degrees of freedom: you can flex or extend it at the humero-ulnar joint and you can rotate your lower arm about its own long axis using the radio-ulnar joint (this latter motion is called supination and pronation). And the wrist also has two degrees of freedom: you can flex or extend it, and you can waggle it back and forth like the late Queen Mother waving. Adding up, the arm, not including the fingers, has $3 + 2 + 2 = 7$ degrees of freedom. Figure 9.2 shows the seven degrees of freedom of the arm. The two dark arms hold 'baseline', or starting, positions, and the seven lighter arms depict the degrees of freedom: on the person's right side are wrist waggle and the three dimensions of shoulder motion; on the other side are wrist extension and the two motions of the elbow.

How many degrees of freedom are there all together in the five fingers of one hand? All five fingers are built on similar plans, though the thumb looks different at first glance. At the base of each digit is a joint that moves with two degrees of freedom (in the case of the thumb, this joint is right up at the wrist). Two distal joints permit just one degree of freedom each. So each digit has four degrees of freedom, for a total of 20 in the hand. But our neural control systems don't seem to use all 20 independently. Some degrees of freedom are hard to decouple, so for instance it takes an effort (well worth it) to learn the Vulcan gesture of greeting, with a V-shaped gap between the middle and ring fingers, or to bend the middle joint of each finger without bending the distal joint, or to place your hand flat on a table and raise, alternately, your index and ring fingers and then your middle and little fingers.

By similar reasoning we can identify and count the degrees of freedom in most sensorimotor systems. Now we are ready to see how unexpected new features can emerge in systems of more than one dimension.

Non-commutativity

One example of a concept that emerges only in higher dimensions is non-commutativity of rotation. What does this mean? Operations or processes are said to *commute* if their order is irrelevant. Ordinary addition of numbers, for instance, is commutative because the order of the addends makes no difference: $3 + 4 = 4 + 3$. You can test this idea at home using piles of oranges—it works for any pair of numbers. Also commutative are one-dimensional rotations: whether you first turn 20 degrees right and then 10 degrees further right, or first 10 degrees and then 20 degrees, you finish up in the same final position, 30 degrees right.

But in three dimensions, rotations don't commute. The upper and lower knights in Fig. 9.3, starting from the same position, undergo the same two rotations but in opposite orders. In the top row, the knight rotates 90 degrees horizontally, about a vertical axis, and then 90 degrees

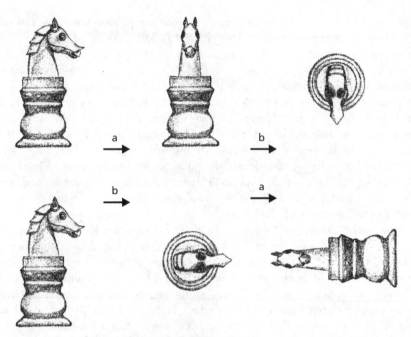

Fig. 9.3 Three-dimensional rotations don't commute: rotation 'a' then 'b' yields a different final position than does 'b' then 'a'.

about a horizontal axis. In the bottom row, the knight undergoes the same rotations about the same axes, but the sequence is reversed. Thanks to non-commutativity, the overall rotations of the two knights and therefore their final positions differ. Figure 9.4 shows that the rotations still don't commute if they are defined from the knight's point of view, in terms of axes that move with him: his order of rotations, first to his right and then nose down or first nose down and then to his right, affects his final position.

Because of non-commutativity, the mathematical techniques for handling translations or one-dimensional rotations don't apply to three-dimensional rotations. Translations or one-dimensional rotations can be represented by vectors or numbers, and can be combined commutatively by adding them together. But three-dimensional rotations call for other, non-commutative algebraic objects and operations. The necessary algebra was developed by mathematicians in the 19th century. Later, in the 1930s, the physicist Paul Dirac marveled that an invention as bizarre as non-commutative algebra had found physical application in quantum mechanics. And essentially the same algebra applies to the motions of the eyes, head, and joints. It is a pleasing thought that quantum physics and sensorimotor biology, the twin pillars of modern science, rest on the same mathematical foundation.

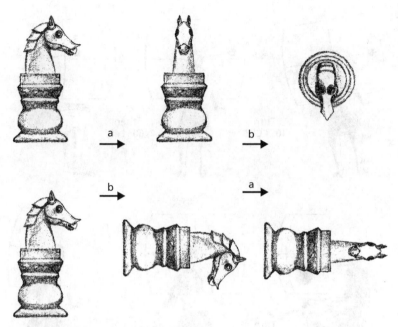

Fig. 9.4 Rotations still don't commute when rotations 'a' and 'b' are defined relative to the turning body itself.

As rotations don't commute, those brain systems that deal with rotary motion—motor circuits that move the eyes, head, and limbs, and sensory and cognitive circuits that handle spatial information—must be capable of non-commutative computation if they are to do their jobs optimally, or even half decently.

Non-commutativity in the brain

Maybe the simplest brain system that deals with rotary motion is the VOR: its sensors in the inner ear measure head rotation and send commands to the eye muscles, counterrotating the eyes when the head turns to prevent the eyeballs turning relative to space. Why does the VOR need non-commutative operators? Imagine you are sitting in a rotary chair, turning through the same two rotations in different orders. Figure 9.5 shows the situation: you are the seated subject. In the figure, you are wearing spandex cycling shorts, though that is not essential to the thought experiment. You begin by looking at a space-fixed target 30 degrees to your left. Then the lights go out, leaving you in pitch darkness, and you begin to rotate. In the upper row, you turn first 10 degrees counterclockwise (CCW) and then 60 degrees left. If you keep your eyes trained on the invisible target, they will finish off pointing 30 degrees right and 5 degrees up,

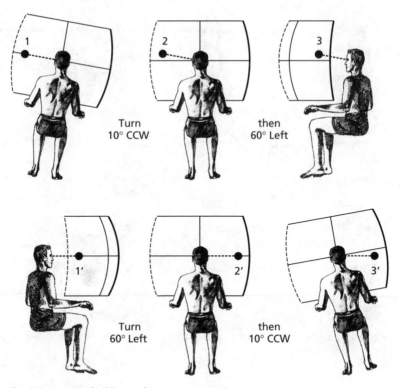

Fig. 9.5 An optimal VOR must be non-commutative.

relative to the straight-ahead position in their sockets. In the lower row, you start with the same eye position and do the same rotations but in the reverse order, first left and then counterclockwise. To stay on target this time, your eyes finish off pointing right and *down*. This thought experiment shows that your VOR, if it is to keep your gaze line on target, must compute different eye-position commands when you undergo the same two rotations in different orders.

When this experiment is actually carried out, the human VOR matches the optimal pattern, keeping the eye on target by driving it to different final positions depending on the order of body rotations.[156] To do this, the circuitry of the VOR must be able to compute the non-commutative geometry of three-dimensional rotations: there must be non-commutative operators in the brain.[157]

And it is not just the VOR that needs these operators. They are essential to almost any brain system that deals with rotation. Spatial memory, for instance, is non-commutative, as you can easily confirm: pick out an object in your surroundings, then rotate your head 90 degrees about two different axes; you will have no trouble correctly picturing the final location of the object relative to your head, even though that location depends on the order of the head turns. And other kinds of information, besides rotary, also call for non-commutative processing, so non-commutativity must be a fairly common feature of sensorimotor systems.

Ascending to higher dimensions

D. A. Robinson's one-dimensional model of the VOR, the one with the integrator that I described in Chapter 6, contains no non-commutative operators because none are needed in one dimension. But then how does Robinson's model apply to the real, three-dimensional reflex, where non-commutative operators are mandatory? In general, how can we extend low-dimensional models to higher dimensions?

The job is difficult because extra dimensions bring so many possibilities. To see the basic problem, imagine that you are a Flatlander, looking at a disk which is the intersection of your world with some solid, three-dimensional object. You know that many solid shapes—a ball, a cylinder, a cone, an ellipsoid, a paraboloid, an egg, and so on—can all look like disks when they intersect your plane. So given the flat disk, how can you guess the solid? In the same way, if you are a neuroscientist, you know that entirely different high-dimensional brain systems would all look the same when you study them in one or two dimensions. So given a low-dimensional model of a neural system, based on low-dimensional data, how can you generalize it so that you improve your chances of matching the real, high-dimensional system in the brain, and of predicting correctly the patterns in high-dimensional data? Common sense is a poor guide, because our unaided intuition doesn't appreciate the strangeness of hyperspace or even three-dimensional space. But there is a way to generalize successfully from low to high dimensions, using optimization.

Taking as our test case Robinson's model of the VOR, the intuitive generalization here is just to triple everything. Turn the eye-velocity command into three eye-velocity commands, for instance horizontal, vertical, and torsional, carried by three channels—or in other words make the eye-velocity command a three-component vector. Turn Robinson's integrator into three integrators, each handling one component of velocity—or in other words make it a vector integrator. And so on. The resulting three-dimensional model is an utter failure, because it is commutative and no commutative mechanism can keep the eye on target when it is put through the rotations from Fig. 9.5.

The problem with the model is Robinson's integrator, which as we saw in Chapter 6 is supposed to compute eye-position commands from eye velocity. One of the surprises that awaits us when we ascend out of Flatland is that in three or more dimensions rotary velocity can't be converted to position by integrating. Introductory calculus books teach that integration turns velocity into position, but these books are talking about translational velocity or one-dimensional rotary velocity. In Chapter 3 I mentioned that the concept of velocity is remarkably sophisticated, so sophisticated that for centuries no one was able to define it, until Augustin Cauchy. But Cauchy's definition doesn't even make sense in the exotic, non-commutative world of three-dimensional rotation. In three dimensions, rotary velocity is defined in another way, as a vector lying along the current axis of spin, its length equal to the rate of spin in degrees per second. The concept is different from translational velocity. It is in some ways analogous—that is why it is called 'velocity'—but it is not identical in all respects, and one difference is that you can't convert it to position by integrating.

You can see this in the pictures of the chess knights in Fig. 9.3 or 9.4. The integral, remember, is just a running sum of the velocity. In the top row of the figure, suppose the knight spins at 90 degrees per second right-ward for 1 s, then at 90 degrees per second downward for 1 s. Then the integral of velocity from start to finish is a vector with horizontal component 90 degrees right and vertical component 90 degrees down. In the bottom row the same velocities are applied in the opposite order. The integral is exactly the same, because an integrator simply accumulates activity like an odometer. It doesn't care whether the knight does the horizontal or the vertical part of the trip first or second. As the integral in the two cases is the same, and the final positions are different, it is clear that position can't be the integral of velocity.

Here is another example of the surprising relation between rotary velocity and position. Place an object on a tabletop in front of you, say a teacup, with its handle toward you (Fig. 9.6). Rotate it 180 degrees horizontally, so now the handle is on the far side. Next turn it 180 degrees vertically in a somersault motion, either up or down, it doesn't matter which. You will see that the cup is now upside down, rotated 180 degrees away from its start position, but it is rotated purely *torsionally*: a clockwise or counterclockwise

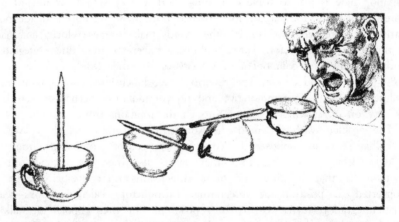

Fig. 9.6 Some people are taken aback by the strange properties of three-dimensional rotations.

flip will put it back where it started. The surprise is that you have changed the cup's torsional position using purely horizontal and vertical rotations, with no torsional velocity. The oddness is concentrated in the second turn. During the first turn, horizontal velocity alters the horizontal orientation of the cup, as you would expect, but in the second turn, the vertical velocity erases the horizontal turn and introduces a torsional one, leaving behind no trace of verticality.

I have met Flatlanders who regard these demonstrations with the knight and the teacup as something like conjuring tricks—deceptions to be exposed. But in fact they are straightforward demonstrations of an interesting and mildly counterintuitive aspect of nature, the non-commutativity of rotations. The teacup story, like the knights', has consequences for eye and limb control because it means that velocity in one dimension, say horizontal, can change the eye's or limb's position in another dimension, vertical or torsional.

In three dimensions, then, you can't compute position from velocity with an integrator. You need a different, non-commutative operator. The details don't matter here; the point is merely that the required operator changes dramatically when we ascend to a higher dimension. If we put the non-commutative operator into our model in place of the integrator, we get a viable VOR that deals perfectly with tasks like those in Fig. 9.5 and correctly predicts other patterns in the three-dimensional data as well. Intuitively, the non-commutative element looks quite different from Robinson's integrator, but from an optimization viewpoint, little has changed. From an optimization viewpoint, Robinson's key insight was that the VOR needs an operator to compute eye-position commands from velocity. In one dimension that operator is an integrator; in three dimensions it is something else, but the idea is the same. If we try to model the VOR in three dimensions based on the letter of Robinson's theory, sending velocity signals through an integrator, we get a model that is unfit for its job. But if we generalize based on the spirit of Robinson's model, using the underlying optimization principle, we are led to the correct three-dimensional analog of his integrator.

So Robinson's integrator isn't really an integrator at all. It is an entity that looks like an integrator to people studying eye control in one dimension. Just as a variety of solid shapes might look like disks in Flatland, so a variety of three-dimensional operators could look like integrators in the one-dimensional VOR. But we can single out the real, three-dimensional operator by considering its role in sensorimotor optimization.

The uses of redundancy

Another principle that arises only in multiple dimensions is redundancy, or systems with more degrees of freedom than they need for some tasks. The arm, for instance, is a redundant mechanism for positioning the hand.

Ignoring the fingers, the hand has six degrees of freedom like any unconstrained rigid body—three degrees of translation and three of rotation. So the arm, with its seven degrees of freedom, has one more that it really needs to position the hand. It can place the hand in any position within arm's length of the shoulder, except for certain awkward back-scratching postures that are unattainable outside Kingsway School playground owing to limited joint ranges, and it does it with one degree of freedom left over. To see where the extra degree has gone, place your hand palm-down on a tabletop, holding it still so that all six of its degrees of freedom are frozen. You will find that without moving your upper body (that is, with arm movement alone) you can still swing your elbow through a small arc. So the six variables describing hand position don't determine the configuration of the arm; a seventh parameter is needed to say where the elbow is along its arc. The arm is kinematically redundant.

But be careful. You can't just count up the degrees of freedom of a mechanism and then declare whether it is fit to perform a particular job, because the degrees of freedom have to be of the right kind. A collapsible telescope or tent pole with eight segments would have seven degrees of freedom, because you would have to specify the amount of extension between each pair of adjacent links to describe the configuration of the whole thing. But a hand stuck on the end of an apparatus like that could not be placed in any arbitrary position, but only translated along a straight line (so the telescope-jointed, prairie townsfolk from a few pages back may not be as menacing as you thought).

Redundancy gives you more than one way to do things. For example, you just found infinitely many different arm postures that allow you to hold your hand in any given position on a table. This kind of surplus freedom brings several advantages. One is obstacle avoidance: if one arm configuration would cause your forearm to graze a high-voltage power line, you can adopt a safer configuration without having to move your hand. Another use of redundancy might be to choose arm configurations where the joints are near the centers of their ranges, so you are better placed for a wide range of subsequent movements, the idea being that holding a joint near the edge of its range is like standing near the edge of the court in tennis. A third advantage of extra freedom is that it provides alternative ways to carry out actions when the usual movements are ruled out owing to injury or fatigue.

Synergies

We normally use our bodies' degrees of freedom only in certain pre-programmed combinations, and we have to make special efforts when we want to program new combinations. It takes special training to learn Vulcan hand gestures. Without lessons it is hard to pat your head and rub your stomach at the same time.

These pre-programmed combinations show up in our limb movements. We can swing our two arms in unison, keeping a constant small separation between our two hands. The coordination is impressive because the motor commands to the two arms are very different. When the right arm moves laterally, pulled by the latissimus dorsi, the left arm moves medially, pulled by the pectoralis muscles. One elbow may be flexing while the other is extending. Muscle activities on the two sides differ, but evidently we have a control module that manages the coordination. This module may have evolved because we need to move our limbs in unison when we use them to shift rigid objects. But we can also move two limbs in mirror symmetry, using another mode of control which we may have developed for activities like swimming.

These modes seem to be quite specific, in the sense that two motion patterns may be in some ways very similar yet one can be performed effortlessly and the other is impossible. For instance you can swing your hands in mirror-image circles in the frontal plane, and you can slowly rotate those circles into the midline plane of the body (so now they are both mirror symmetric and in unison). But if you swing your hands in circles *in unison* in the frontal plane, you can't rotate those circles into the midline plane without losing your coordination, presumably because then the motions don't have the sort of unison that is compatible with holding a rigid object. You can rotate your hands or your feet in the midline plane in unison but with a 180 degree phase shift, as in dog paddling or running. But if you try to rotate your hands out of phase in the frontal plane, your circles get sloppy.

The lesson is that much of our motor control works with pre-programmed modules that activate certain especially useful motions. Our motor plans don't so much play on the keyboard of the muscles as load prefabricated player-piano rolls. These pre-programmed patterns are called synergies.

If we want to understand synergies, the best approach, as usual, is to start simple. And as often happens, the simplest and best-understood cases involve the brain systems that control the eyes. The concepts we find in these simple cases generalize widely.

Donders' law

We have seen that the eye has three degrees of freedom: horizontal, vertical, and torsional. Three degrees of freedom are required for some visual tasks, but for others they are redundant. All three are needed to keep the retinal image stable during head rotation, the job of the VOR, because the eye's motion has to oppose the head's in all dimensions. But it is another story when the task is to aim the line of sight. Here the controlled variable—the direction of the gaze line—has only two degrees of freedom. To see this, imagine yourself sitting at the center of a large globe made of glass; then you can specify your gaze direction with just two numbers, namely the longitude and latitude of the point where your line of sight intersects the globe. So when you aim your gaze line at an object, you are using an eye with three degrees of freedom to control a two-dimensional variable. For this task the eye is kinematically redundant.

So in theory, whenever you look at anything you have a choice among infinitely many different eye positions: you can twist your eye x degrees around the line of sight, where x is any number, without displacing your gaze from its target (Fig. 9.7). What does the brain do with the extra, torsional degree of freedom? It implements Donders' law, which was discovered in the nineteenth century by F.C. Donders.[158] He was a physiologist, famous enough to be commemorated on a Dutch stamp in 1935, almost 50 years after his death.

Donders' law says that *we always select the same eye position every time we look in a given direction.* The eye's angle of twist about its line of sight is always the same for any one gaze direction. All other twist angles are illegal.

You can verify Donders' law as he himself did if you can form persistent afterimages. In a dimly lit room, burn a linear or straight-edged afterimage into your retina by staring at a bright line or edge—a fluorescent tube, or the light stripes between Venetian blinds, or the edge of a bright window (don't, obviously, look near the sun). Then look around the room, being careful to keep your head still. The angle of your afterimage, seen against the perpendicular lines of the room, makes visible to you the twist of your own eye about its line of sight. If your afterimage fades, you can refresh it by blinking. You should find that without moving your head you can't, by any act of will, make the afterimage rotate clockwise or counterclockwise. Your ocular torsion isn't under your voluntary control, but is dictated by the unconscious Donders mechanisms in your brain. The afterimage will twist slightly as you look in different directions, but for any one gaze direction it is always the same, at least as far as you can tell. Precise measurements with magnetic search coils confirm that the eye's

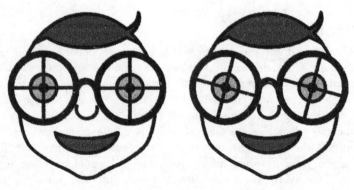

Fig. 9.7 Ocular torsion.

angle of twist is always the same in any one gaze direction to within about a degree.

The general idea behind Donders' law is that the brain controls redundant degrees of freedom so as to make them a function of the non-redundant ones. This is a widely applicable concept. Analogs of Donders' law hold for many, and probably for all, sensorimotor systems. The head obeys a version of Donders' law during spontaneous eye–head gaze shifts: whenever you face in any one direction, you always adopt the same head orientation. The hand, too, obeys Donders' law at least roughly during some tasks. During straight-arm pointing, it adopts only one hand position for any one pointing direction. For the head and hand, Donders' law is less rigidly enforced than for the eye: you can voluntarily twist your neck or arm into almost any angle you like. But the default, automatic pattern of head and arm control obeys Donders' law during spontaneous gaze shifts and straight-arm pointing.

The law has surprising repercussions for motor control. For instance, an attractive idea is that we control our movement in a way that always takes the shortest path to our goal. But in a redundant system, Donders' law rules out some short paths. Imagine an eye looking back and forth

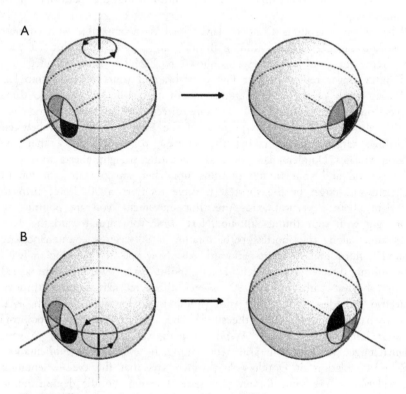

Fig. 9.8 Different eye rotations can cause the same change in gaze direction.

between two targets, say two objects in a horizontal plane, 60 degrees apart, as in Fig. 9.8. The eye has many possible paths. It can move between the targets by rotating 60 degrees horizontally about a vertical axis, as in Fig. 9.8A. It can achieve the same gaze shift by rotating 180 degrees about a forward-pointing axis that bisects the angle between the targets, as in Fig. 9.8B. The 180 degree rotation seems an unlikely choice, because it involves flipping the eye upside down, but it shows that the pure horizontal rotation isn't the only option. In fact, there are infinitely many possible axes: the eye could rotate about any axis in the plane bisecting the angle between the target directions.

The eye rotation is smallest, or in other words takes the shortest path, when the axis is orthogonal to both the initial and final gaze directions. In the case of two targets in the horizontal plane, for example, the axis of the shortest path is vertical. As the axis tilts away from orthogonal, the size of the rotation you need increases. So if your brain wanted to aim your gaze line using the smallest possible eye rotations it would always choose the rotation axis that is orthogonal to the initial and final gaze directions. But it does not do this. Instead, your axes tip slightly but systematically away from the shortest-path axes. Evidently the brain cares about something other than minimizing the path length of saccades.

What it cares about is Donders' law, which is incompatible with shortest paths. You can see this by running through an exercise where you let your hand represent your turning eye, as shown in Fig. 9.9. Your extended arm and index finger represent your line of sight, and your cocked thumb lets you keep track of torsional rotations, about the sight line. Choose three targets, one straight ahead of you, one directly to your right, and one directly above your head. The purpose of the exercise is to point between the three targets, always taking the shortest path, and show that the motion violates Donders' law. Begin by pointing straight ahead with your palm vertical and your thumb pointing up. Then sweep your arm toward the rightward target by the shortest possible rotation, a 90 degree turn to the right about a vertical axis. After this movement, you are pointing to your right with your thumb still up. Next swing your arm toward the overhead target along the shortest path, rotating it 90 degrees counterclockwise around a horizontal, forward–backward axis. Now you are pointing up with your thumb directed to the left. Finally, point back toward straight ahead by the shortest path, rotating 90 degrees about an axis running through your two shoulders. Notice that your thumb is no longer sticking up, as it was when last you pointed at the straight-ahead target, but is now pointing to your left. Taking always the shortest path, you have returned to your original target but with your arm, representing the eye, in a new orientation. This is a violation of Donders' law, which says that the eye's orientation must always be the same for any one gaze direction. So the demonstration shows that it is impossible both to follow Donders' law and always to take

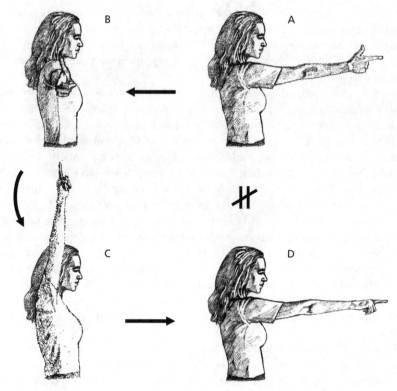

Fig. 9.9 Donders' law rules out shortest paths.

the shortest paths between pointing directions. Any rotary system must choose one (or neither) of these strategies. The brain systems that aim the gaze line choose Donders' law.

Why Donders?

Donders' law can be understood on optimization grounds. Why do saccades and head and arm movements follow this law instead of taking the shortest paths to their targets? One reason is revealed if we continue the pointing demonstration we used just now to show that Donders' law and shortest paths are incompatible. Choose three targets, one straight ahead, one to your right, and one straight above you. Begin the exercise by pointing at the straight-ahead target with your thumb pointing up. Swing to the rightward target, to the overhead target, and back to straight ahead, always taking the shortest path, as in the earlier demonstration. Now your thumb is pointing left. It has rotated 90 degrees counterclockwise from its original position. Swing once more through the cycle of three targets, and now your thumb is turned 180 degrees counterclockwise. After another cycle, the thumb is turned 270 degrees, and the arm position is becoming awkward. By relentlessly taking the shortest path, you accumulate torsion, twisting your arm further and further. If you did the same to your eye, you would twist it on your optic nerve like a soap-on-a-rope. This may be one reason that eye, head, and hand reject shortest paths in favor of Donders' law.

Here is one piece of evidence that Donders' law serves in part to prevent torsional accumulation. Your head obeys Donders' law when you look around you with spontaneous eye–head gaze shifts, and when you look between several targets in response to randomly ordered verbal commands (look left, look up, and so on). But it breaks Donders' law, and actually tends toward shortest-path movements, when you are asked to look back and forth repeatedly between two targets.[159] Why? The likely reason is that there is no danger of torsional accumulation if you take the shortest path back and forth between two targets, because each movement undoes the previous one. Apparently the head-control centers are clever enough to see this, so they switch toward a more efficient, shortest-path mode. This mode of action doesn't seem to establish itself gradually, over a few cycles of movement. Instead it is present in the very first movement between the two targets, which means that it is the intention to cycle, rather than the cycling itself, that alters the motor pattern.

Another advantage of Donders' law of the eye may be that it simplifies spatial vision. If you see an object, then the retinal image alone tells you its direction relative to your eye. But often you need to know where things are relative to your head or your torso and limbs, for instance when you want to reach for them or move to avoid them. For this, you need information about eye position. If an object lies 10 degrees right relative to your eye, where is it relative to your head? If your eye is turned 30 degrees right in your head, the object is 40 degrees right; if your eye is turned 30 degrees left, the object is 20 degrees left. In general you need to know the eye's position in all three dimensions. But Donders' law may reduce the information you need to specify eye position, because it removes the third degree of freedom. It makes the torsional component of eye position a function of the horizontal and vertical components, so if you know the horizontal and vertical angles, you know everything.

A problem with this idea, though, is that Donders' law doesn't hold exactly. Ocular torsion isn't exactly the same every time you look in a given direction. It varies overs a range of a degree or two, so the third dimension isn't in fact entirely removed. Either the brain needs information about ocular torsion after all, or it must be prepared to accept the consequences of ignoring it. I will return to this question in Chapter 10.

Donders' law, you may have noticed, says that the eye adopts a unique orientation for each gaze direction, but it doesn't say *which* orientation. The quantitative rule is given by Listing's law.

Listing's law

Johann Benedict Listing was a mathematician, a friend and colleague of Carl Friedrich Gauss and a professor of mathematical physics at Göttingen University at a time when Göttingen was the Olympus of math. He apparently formulated his law of eye motion—the most famous, best-studied, and most misunderstood of all motor synergies—based on pure geometric esthetics. He never tried to test whether it was correct, nor did he publish anything on the subject. It was Hermann von Helmholtz who named Listing's law and verified it by measuring the tilts of afterimages.[160] The law is notoriously complicated to state.

Listing's law says, first of all, that there is a special plane, fixed in the head, called Listing's plane; the plane is 'imaginary' in the sense that it is invisible and can't be detected by any known anatomical investigation, but it is real enough, and can be located by methods I will describe in a moment. There is also a special eye position called the primary position, usually close to what we would intuitively call straight ahead, in which the gaze line is at right angles to Listing's plane. Then Listing's law says that *the eye adopts only those orientations that can be reached from primary position by a single rotation about an axis in Listing's plane.*

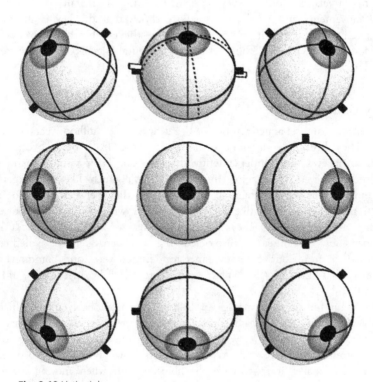

Fig. 9.10 Listing's law.

In Fig. 9.10, Listing's plane is the plane of the paper, and the eye at the center is in the primary position. All the eye orientations drawn with solid lines accord with Listing's law, because they can be reached from the primary position by rotating about axes (the black lines) in Listing's plane. But the position drawn with dashed lines at the top center violates Listing's law, because the rotation to that orientation from the primary position has its axis (the white line) tilted out of Listing's plane. I said that Listing's plane can't be detected by examining the anatomy of the skull; it is manifest in the control of the eyes. You can find it only by measuring eye rotations and computing the common plane of their axes.

When you obey Listing's law, you automatically obey Donders' law: every time you look in any given direction, you always use the same eye orientation.[161] In Fig. 9.10, for example, the eyes drawn with solid and dashed lines at top center both point the gaze line in the same upward direction, but only the eye drawn in solid lines fits Listing's law.

We can express Listing's law more simply if we define ocular 'torsion' as rotation about an axis outside Listing's plane. Then Listing's law says that *ocular torsion is always zero*: the eye's separation from the primary position involves no torsional rotation.

The law holds when we fixate targets, look between targets, or track moving targets, as long as we hold the head still. It fails during rolling head movements and in sleep. Its failure shows that the law is neural and not purely mechanical: it is not imposed on the eye by the anatomy of its muscles or bony socket, but reflects the neural signals that activate the muscles.

Why Listing?

Chameleons are separated from us by at least 200 million years of evolution. They live in a different oculomotor world from ours, because they rotate their eyes more independently than we do. Their visual experience is hard for us even to imagine (probably it isn't much like our experience watching a split movie screen, because we just flick between the two image fields; maybe it is more like feeling the world with two hands). But alien as they are, chameleons obey Listing's law just as we do.[162] I don't know whether our two lineages discovered the law separately or whether we inherited it from our common ancestor. Either way, our common bond suggests that Listing's law plays some crucial role in vision and eye control.[163]

The main functional advantage of Listing's law is probably motor efficiency. The law ensures that all gaze shifts toward and away from the primary position take the shortest path. We have seen that it is impossible always to take the shortest path and still follow Donders' law, but it *is* possible—and Listing's law makes it so—to take the shortest path when moving toward or away from the primary gaze direction. This way, the eye, wherever it looks, always stays as close as possible to the primary position. Of all the infinitely many orientations compatible with any gaze direction, the eye adopts the one whose three-dimensional rotary separation from the primary position is as small as possible. Why is this useful? It may reduce muscle work, as proposed in the 19th century by Adolph Fick and Wilhelm Wundt.[164, 165] And it is another instance of the center-court principle I mentioned a few pages back as one of the uses of redundancy; staying as close as possible to the primary position carries the same advantages as staying near the center of the court in tennis, permitting fast and flexible responses to unpredictable targets that may appear from any direction.

Donders and Listing in hyperspace

Undoubtedly there are, still waiting to be discovered, many higher-dimensional analogs of Donders' and Listing's laws. Donders' law confines the eye, for some tasks, to a two-dimensional subset of the three-dimensional space of all eye positions. There is probably a suite of analogous laws that confine the arm, for some of its tasks, to various subsets of the seven-dimensional space of all its possible orientations. Or, generalizing the idea slightly, there may be laws that confine the positions *and velocities* of the arm joints to some subset of the fourteen-dimensional space of all possible positions and velocities; and more abstract generalizations are also possible. Whatever their form, these sorts of Donders' law analogs are one kind of constraint that will simplify our descriptions of the brain.

Higher-dimensional learning

Learning multidimensional operations requires no new mechanisms beyond those we have considered. All the strange, high-dimensional properties like non-commutativity and synergy arise automatically. For instance a three-dimensional VOR network, driven by an error signal coding retinal slip, would automatically develop non-commutativity because non-commutative operators are waiting in the deepest optima of the energy landscape.

This point is crucial because it shows that some sensorimotor concepts do generalize to higher dimensions. It is true that high-dimensional systems bring all sorts of surprises. They call for new concepts like non-commutativity. They alter Robinson's integrator to the point where it isn't quite an integrator any more. But often the same optimization principle, for instance minimizing retinal slip, that works in one dimension automatically yields the exotic new features in the higher-dimensional case.

Mounting complexity

For the last few chapters I have been charting the three-fold path—the approach to brain function based on computers and sensorimotor optimization.

How far can this path take us? It has worked well so far, though admittedly on simpler subsystems of the brain. It has been easy enough to work out optimization principles and plausible error signals for the VOR and for fast eye and arm movements. Now I take the next step, applying the same methods to a system of greater complexity. My point will be that the trend is encouraging—as sensorimotor systems grow in complexity, their detailed behavior becomes impossible to predict intuitively but the optimization principles remain simple or even the same.

I will illustrate this idea using eye–head coordination. This is a high-dimensional problem. The two eyes each rotate with three degrees of freedom, the head rotates and translates with six degrees of freedom, and the visual target can be anywhere in three-dimensional space, for a total of fifteen degrees of freedom in all. We're not in Flatland anymore. But this sensorimotor system provides a clear example of the explanatory and predictive power of simple optimization ideas.

Eye–head coordination

When the eye and head combine forces to transport the gaze line, the logistics become complex. For one thing, the eye is quicker than the head: it reorients faster when an interesting object appears in the visual periphery. Like a gunner in a Star Wars-style fighter craft, the eye pivots rapidly to the visual target and locks on, hanging almost stationary in space while the head maneuvers more slowly into position. Several laboratories have charted how eye–head gaze shifts unfold in the horizontal plane.[166-170] The eye usually starts moving first, followed a few milliseconds later by the head. Normally, the VOR would respond to the head rotation by counter-rotating the eye, but in a large eye–head gaze shift the VOR is switched off. From an optimization viewpoint this makes perfect sense, as the function of the VOR is to hold the gaze point stationary in space, and during a gaze shift you don't want a stationary gaze point. With the VOR off, the head can help transport the gaze line. The eye reaches its objective while the head is still *en route*. At this moment the VOR switches back on and holds the eye on target as the head completes its motion. The maneuver demands impressive accuracy and split-second timing, as the VOR may have to switch off and then on again within a tenth of a second. And it all works without visual guidance, because vision is too slow. In the lab you can record and display, as different colored symbols on a computer screen, the trajectories of the gaze point and of the target relative to the head, which is also continuously moving because the head is turning. When you rerun the maneuver in slow motion, you witness the stirring spectacle of the eye swooping in on its target like a falcon on a sparrow, or a dog on a frisbee. But the whole complex sequence of events is just what you would expect of an optimized system that is trying to get the eye as quickly as possible to its target and then hold it there.

A surprising prediction emerges when we consider how an optimized system for eye–head coordination would handle Listing's law. In accordance with that law, you want your eye to end up with near-zero torsion when the gaze shift is complete, that is, when the head comes to rest. But then how do you aim the eye? Of course you want to point the line of sight at the target, but what value do you want for the eye's torsional angle in its socket at the moment when it reaches the target? Zero degrees, to fit Listing's law? No, because at this point the head is still moving, and the VOR, now switched back on again, is rotating the eye in its socket horizontally, vertically, and torsionally to hold it steady in space. The VOR doesn't preserve Listing's law (if it did, it couldn't properly stabilize the retinal image during torsional head motion), so if your eye obeyed the law at the moment it attained the target it would no longer do so by the time the head stopped moving. So your short-lead burst neurons have to drive your eye to a non-zero torsional position that has been carefully chosen so that, when the head completes its turn, the eye will land back at zero torsion. The burst neurons have to wind up the eye's torsion, in some cases to quite extreme angles, over 15 degrees, and then let the VOR wind it back down again. In other words the system should break Listing's law in a dramatic fashion during the movement so that it can obey the law again when the movement is complete.

Simulations of the optimized model predict large violations of Listing's law during gaze shifts involving torsional head motion. One such task is illustrated in Fig. 9.11. The subject starts out in the position marked A, with the head turned 30 degrees counterclockwise, or left-ear down, and the eyes directed 20 degrees down in the head, looking at a laser spot. The spot jumps 20 degrees to the left, and the subject makes a rolling eye–head movement to refixate it, ending up in position C. According to the optimized model, the eye should reach its final orientation in space

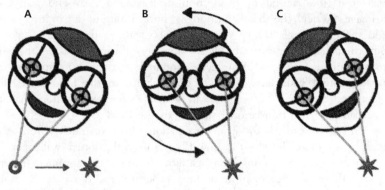

Fig. 9.11 Torsional saccade.

when the head is still turning, so relative to the head, the eye should twist, as shown in B. This is a daring prediction because the torsion amounts to 15 degrees, which is an almost unheard of violation of Listing's law.

When real people perform this task, they behave as predicted by the optimized model, generating the largest torsional eye movements ever seen in healthy humans.[171] Like the spectacled boy in the figure, they obey Listing's law before and after the gaze shift, but during the movement they show almost grotesque angles of eye-in-head torsion, often more than 15 degrees, as predicted. Typically, the eye spins about the line of sight at up to 200 degrees per second for 80 ms or so and then unwinds back to near-zero torsion over about 200 ms.

Underlying these movements is a sophisticated control system, but everything in it follows from a few optimization principles: look at the target and stabilize the retinal image as quickly as possible, and when the movement is over, make sure the eye obeys Listing's law, so that it is positioned near the center of the court ready for a quick response to the next target. The analysis demonstrates the power of optimization ideas to render neural systems comprehensible. For another example, we turn from gaze transport to gaze stabilization.

Vestibular light and magic

In a freely moving animal in three-dimensional space, the VOR faces challenges akin to those of computer animation. The top row of Fig. 9.12 shows how, without the VOR, the retinal image would slip during horizontal, vertical, and torsional head rotations, also called yaw, pitch, and roll.[172] In each panel we see, projected onto the retina, the image of a field of spots, say the night sky or speckled wallpaper. Streaks show how the retinal images of these points smear out as the head rotates. The pattern of smear lines is called optical flow. The VOR works on the principle that eye rotation can create a pattern of optical flow that cancels the flow caused by head motion, leaving a clear and stable retinal image. When the head motion is pure rotation, an optimal VOR would make the eye's rotary velocity equal -1 times the head's.

But what happens when the head translates through space rather than just spinning in one spot? Your eyes, mounted in their bony sockets, can't translate around your face. Their motion relative to the head is restricted to rotation. So the VOR's job is to generate the eye rotation that best compensates for the translational motion of the head.

Optical flows caused by head translation differ markedly from those caused by rotation. If you run toward a wall with dotted wallpaper, you see a looming, or expanding, flow pattern. If you carry a camera in front of you with its shutter open in a time exposure, the dots on the wallpaper will smear out into lines radiating from a center which is the point of

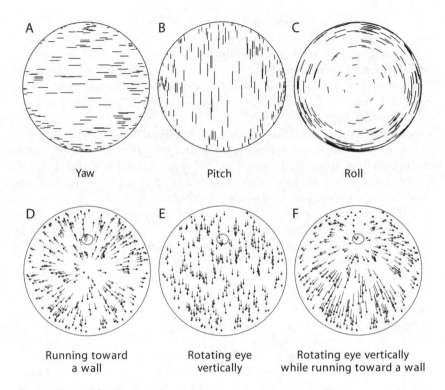

Fig. 9.12 Optical flows.

imminent impact (Fig. 9.12D illustrates the flow, with arrows to mark the direction). No *rotation* of the head could produce this radial flow, and no eye rotation can cancel it. So no eye rotation can perfectly stabilize the retinal image when the head translates.

Another feature that appears only in translational flows is parallax, meaning that nearby objects smear out more than distant ones. Think of the view out the window of a train that is speeding along a straight track. Nearby rail ties and trees whiz by while distant hills creep slowly. The sun, or the moon and stars, seem to keep perfect pace with the train, except when you go round a bend, that is, when the train rotates. Walt Disney worked hard to simulate parallax in his animated films using the technique of multiplaning, where foreground and background objects are drawn on separate clear sheets which can be slid about independently. You can see the effect at the beginning of *Beauty and the Beast*, when the 'camera' moves—translates—up from the forest toward the Beast's castle. What does parallax mean for the VOR? As rotation causes no parallax, no eye rotation can cancel the parallax caused by head translation.

So how do we manage to see while we translate? The problem is especially pressing for pigeons, chickens, and some other birds. With their eyes on the sides of their heads, they see the visual world stream across their retinas whenever they walk. The solution they have developed, or inherited from the dinosaurs, is to hold the head stationary in space while the body walks forward beneath it, and then snap the head forward very quickly to begin the cycle again. With this gait, the head is stationary most of the time; the periods of retinal-image slip are compressed into the brief intervals while the head snaps forward.

Ballerinas use a similar head-snapping technique to stay on their feet during spins, but for retinal-image stabilization during locomotion, mammals, including lateral-eyed ones like rabbits, have rejected this solution, maybe because mammalian heads and necks are somehow mechanically unsuited to constant jerking. In any case, humans and other primates and probably cats (the only species that have been thoroughly tested) take a different approach. As it is impossible to stabilize the entire retinal image using eye rotation, we stabilize part of it. However the head is moving, it is always possible to rotate the eye in a way that stabilizes the image of any particular point in space. We choose the eye rotation that stabilizes the visual target, or at least that part of the target whose image falls on the fovea, the small central patch of retina, densely connected with the brain, that is specialized for high-acuity vision.[34, 173, 174]

This approach involves some complex geometry, as the required eye rotation depends not only on head velocity, as in the rotary case, but also on target location. To maintain fixation on a spot on the ceiling as you translate forward, you have to rotate your eyes upward; to fixate a spot on the floor you rotate your eyes down. What this would do to a translational, looming optical flow is shown in Fig. 9.12. In panel D, a moving observer has directed the fovea (the small ellipse in the picture) vertically away from straight ahead: the uncompensated optical flow in the foveal region is upward. The VOR responds with a vertical eye rotation that, were the head stationary, would generate the optical flow seen in panel E. So the net optical flow is the sum of D and E, shown in part F: the VOR has succeeded in canceling the retinal slip over the fovea (compare the tiny specks in the foveal ellipse in panel F with the longer radial streaks at the same location in panel D). Over the lower part of the field, the eye rotation aggravates the retinal image slip, but this region is less important than the fovea.

We need complex processing also to cope with parallax, because eye velocity has to vary inversely with the distance to the visual target. And indeed, when you translate, your eyes rotate faster when the target is closer and slower when it is far away, just as they must to stabilize the target image. To see this effect, look out of a nearby window with crossbars or open blinds and bob up and down. If you fix your attention on the distant scene outside you will find that its image remains clear and fixed on your fovea as you oscillate vertically, while the bars of the window are not fixed: they slide down relative to your gaze point when you rise upward and they slide up when you sink down. But if you shift your attention to the window bars, then they will remain stable and the distant world will oscillate, up when you move up, down when you move down. All these adjustments for target direction and distance can be driven by the vestibular sensors, with no help from the eyes, because they also occur in the dark and too quickly to be guided by vision.[34, 173, 175-177]

So the VOR is tuned to the location of the visual target. But how can your VOR keep track of the target's location without seeing it? The puzzle is that your vestibular sensors can monitor head motion at extremely short latency but cannot themselves see where the target is. Other senses, such as vision, hearing, and touch, can tell you where the target is, but they work too slowly to track its location, relative to your body, when you are moving fast. The solution is to rely on these slow senses as long as your head is stationary or moving slowly. During rapid body movements, you store the most recently available sensory estimate of target location relative to your head, and use fast vestibular information about head motion to compute how that location is changing.

If you see a clock 5 meters straight ahead of you and then the lights go out and you translate 1 meter forward and turn 90 degrees to the left, your vestibular target tracker computes that the clock must now be 4 meters to your right. If your otoliths say that you are translating steadily forward at 1 m s^{-1}, your tracker computes that all objects in your environment are streaming backwards, relative to you, at the same speed. If your semicircular canals say that you are rotating to the right, the tracker computes that all objects are circulating in the opposite direction along horizontal circles centered on your axis of rotation (a vertical line running through your head): objects in front of you are translating left, while objects to your left, behind you, and to your right translate backward, rightward, and forward.

The computations within the vestibular tracker are essentially the same as those involved in computer animation. I mentioned that Walt Disney Studios simulated parallax using multiplaning in the opening seconds of *Beauty and the Beast*. But multiplaning only roughly mimics parallax because it uses only a small, finite number of sliding planes. Perfect parallax is achieved by computer animation, as in the ballroom scene where Belle and the Beast dance and Mrs Potts sings the title track. Here, a geometric description of an elliptical ballroom, complete with pillars, chandelier, and windows, sits inside a computer. A simulated movie camera is placed into the ballroom, and the program computes what the room looks like through the camera. As the camera glides and turns, the program computes the optical flow: approaching objects loom larger, receding objects contract, and nearby pillars or chandeliers sweep past quickly while the far windows are nearly stationary, as long as the simulated camera is not rotating.

Here the stored geometric data about the layout of the ballroom are analogous to visual, auditory, and proprioceptive data about initial object locations; the trajectory of the camera is analogous to the head motion sensed by the vestibular organs; and the computation of the resulting image flow corresponds to the processing in the vestibular tracker. A simulated VOR built on these principles does a good job of predicting real human eye movements during natural head motion. This doesn't prove that the brain uses the same equations as Walt Disney Studios, but it does show that the VOR's networks implement something closely equivalent to those equations.

But the brain's job is more complex because it works with two cameras. Because the two eyes are separated in the head, we have to turn them at different rates when the head moves. In experiments, the match is very close between optimal eye speeds and the behavior of real humans. Theoretically, an optimal VOR would turn the eyes not just at different speeds but also about different axes. This prediction hasn't yet been tested, but I would be surprised if it weren't soon verified. An optimal VOR should operate with five degrees of freedom, so our ocular repertoire probably rivals that of chameleons. Of the six possible degrees of freedom of the two eyes, the only one we don't need for an optimal VOR is disjunctive vertical motion, one eye moving up and the other down.

Revealed in all its degrees of freedom, the VOR threatens to surpass understanding. The equations relating its fifteen dimensions are complex and nonlinear. Their implications can be drawn out only by computer simulation. But the same optimization principle that governs the VOR in the simplest case—one-dimensional, purely rotary motion—also explains most of the complex higher-dimensional behavior. A suitably adaptive network, driven by an error signal coding retinal slip, would automatically learn to cope with looming optical flow, parallax, binocularity, and non-commutativity. Once again, proliferating degrees of freedom introduce new concepts and complexities, but from an optimization viewpoint little may be changed.

Chapter 10

The flow of information

Information is in some ways like so much water that has to be pumped from place to place in the brain. To move more information you need a stronger pump or a bigger pipe. And contaminants can reduce the amount of useful information that arrives at the far end. It was an American engineer, Claude Shannon, who in the late 1940s managed to define, in a precise way, the concept of information. He defined the unit of information, called

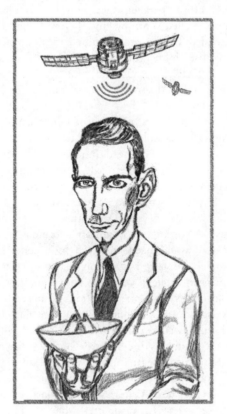

Fig. 10.1 Claude Shannon developed the theory of information and communication.

the bit, which I mentioned in Chapters 2 and 3, and he derived mathematical formulae for estimating the number of bits in a signal and for quantifying how signals are contaminated by noise. Here I take a deeper look at his ideas and their implications for the brain, though I will still just brush the surface of his theory. It is easy, or at least I find it easy, to forget about information flow and noise, to write computer simulations of the brain that are noise-free, where digital signals glide through cyberspace without degrading at all. But the real brain battles noise at every turn, and many aspects of its function make sense only when we realize that they are attempts to function optimally in the presence of noise.

Inside information

Shannon's concept of information is best understood by considering its flip-side, the concept of uncertainty. The two ideas are closely related because you need more information to resolve more uncertainty. In fact the information you need to answer a question equals the uncertainty that exists before the answer arrives. Shannon called his uncertainty concept *entropy*, because of certain parallels between his formula and the formula for another quantity called entropy in thermodynamics. Apparently the name was recommended by the great mathematical physicist, game theorist, and computer scientist John von Neumann, who said it would give Shannon an edge in debate because no one knows what entropy is. But the thermodynamic parallel doesn't help me much, so I will stick to the term *uncertainty*.

Uncertainty arises when events are governed by chance. When you flip a coin you don't know which side will land up, though you do know that there is a 50 per cent chance of heads and a 50 per cent chance of tails (assuming the coin is minted symmetrically, and ignoring unlikely outcomes like the coin balancing on its edge). So you are uncertain about the outcome of the toss. If you are throwing a die, you are even more uncertain because now there are six possible outcomes rather than two. Can we quantify uncertainty? According to Shannon's formula it is the number of yes-or-no questions you would need answered to become certain. If I toss a coin that you know to be fair, but I don't show you the result, you can work it out by getting a straight yes-or-no answer to just one question, for instance 'Is it heads?'. As just one question is needed, your uncertainty, before the question is answered, amounts to 1 bit. This is as far as I took the matter when I first discussed bits in Chapter 3.

More precisely, uncertainty is the number of questions you need *on average* to become certain. Suppose that you want to know who the next person through your door will be, and that you know the odds: there is a one-half chance that the next visitor will be Mary, a one-quarter chance that it will be Peter and a one-quarter chance that it will be Paul. Obviously no single yes-or-no question can settle the matter in all cases, because there are three possibilities. But if we run this scenario over and over again, you can resolve your uncertainty with one-and-a-half questions on average. For instance, your first question each time could be 'Is it a woman?'. Half the time, the answer will be 'yes', in which case your enquiry is over; you know your visitor is Mary. But half the time, the answer will be 'no', in which case you will need to ask a second question, such as 'Is it Peter?'. On a typical run of a hundred repetitions, in fifty cases you will ask one question and in the other fifty cases two questions, for a total of one hundred and fifty questions in a hundred trials. On average, then, you will need one-and-a-half questions, which means that your uncertainty each time you face this scenario is 1.5 bits. By similar reasoning you can show that the uncertainty before every toss of a fair die is about 2.58 bits, though in this case the optimal sequence of questions is less intuitive.

Suppose I throw an unfair coin, one where the likelihood of landing heads is 75 per cent and the likelihood of tails is 25 per cent. Then my uncertainty before each throw comes to just 0.81 bit. Of course I can't pose 0.81 yes-or-no questions, but if you toss the coin a hundred times and record the results, then for an average set of a hundred tosses, I will need about eighty-one questions to sort out which of the hundred tosses yielded heads and which yielded tails, if I choose my questions wisely (and as with the die, it takes some thought to figure out what those questions should be). So an unfair coin toss contains less information than a fair toss. Another way to see this is to notice that tossing an entirely unfair coin, say one that always lands heads, involves no uncertainty at all. The slightly unfair coin is a step along the road to complete unfairness, so it makes sense that its uncertainty should be intermediate between 1 and 0 bits. If you were betting even money against a coin tosser, and you knew the probabilities of the coin, you couldn't gain any advantage if the coin were fair, but if it were unfair you could accumulate winnings by exploiting your diminished uncertainty.

The point is that you can reduce uncertainty by reducing the number of possible outcomes, which is why tossing a coin involves less uncertainty than tossing a die. And more surprisingly, you can also reduce uncertainty by leaving the number of outcomes the same but making some of them less likely—that is why tossing an unfair coin involves less uncertainty than tossing a fair coin. Both mechanisms are probably used in the brain. They may, for instance, repair the gap in my account from last chapter of the function of Donders' law. I said that the law simplifies spatial vision because it removes a dimension. It makes the torsional dimension of eye position calculable from the horizontal and vertical dimensions, so the brain need only keep track of two components of eye motion. Strictly speaking, though, the torsional dimension is not removed but merely restricted, so eye-position information must be three-dimensional after all. But the restriction, and the fact that eye positions become less and less likely the more they depart from Donders' law, reduces the amount of information that has to be transmitted about eye position. So Donders' law is a matter of reducing not precisely the dimensions but rather the uncertainty of ocular positioning, so that less information has to be pumped to the visual processors.

Information overload

One of the main reasons we make eye movements at all is to solve a problem of information flow. We make saccades to bring the images of interesting objects onto the fovea, for high-acuity vision. Our whole visual field apart from the tiny disk that falls on the fovea is seen poorly, not because it is out of focus, but because the retinal ganglion cells there are widely spaced. Away from the fovea, the retina is like a computer screen with too few pixels. Normally we don't notice how bad our peripheral vision is, but if you fix your gaze *here* and try to read on without moving your eyes, you will see that only the nearest neighboring words are legible. This shows why we make 100 000 saccades a day.

We wouldn't have to make so many saccades if our foveae were larger. Why not make the fovea as large as the whole retina? Then our entire visual field would be seen in high resolution. We could read a book or survey a scene without ever moving our eyes. But we would have a new problem. If the whole retina were as densely innervated with ganglion cells as the fovea is, the total number of those cells would be increased about a hundred-fold. It has been estimated that a fifth of all the information pouring into the brain arrives through the eyes, so a hundred-fold increase in retinal input would magnify the brain's total sensory inflow some twenty-fold, which might overwhelm us. Natural selection therefore rejected big foveae and opted for a fast and accurate saccadic system to aim small foveae at targets of interest in order to achieve a manageable flow of information through the optic pipeline.

To get some quantitative notion of the advantage, consider that the human optic nerve contains about one million axons, which is like representing the entire visual field with just a million pixels. That sounds pitiful compared with the three million pixels we demand in our digital cameras, but it is actually not bad given that most of our pixels are tiny ones clustered tightly in and around the fovea. Relatively few, coarse pixels tile the periphery. Some robots are built on the same principle, with heterogeneous foveated retinas in their mobile eyes.

Small foveae also let us avoid other sensorimotor problems. If our foveae were as large as our retinas, the number of nerve fibers exiting the eye would have to increase a hundred-fold. The optic nerve at the back of the eyeball would be about as thick as the eye itself, and might hamper its mobility. (Even with huge foveae, the eyes would still have to move. Saccades wouldn't be needed so much, but we would still need the VOR, optokinesis, and pursuit to hold images stationary on the retina, unless our visual processors were redesigned to cope better with moving images. Even saccades would still be needed sometimes to bring new objects into the visual field, as when you hear someone sneaking up behind you and turn around to look. During sustained head rotations, as well, we would need saccades to recenter our eyes periodically when the VOR brought them to their mechanical limits.)

Large foveae would also mean large blind spots. Our eyes, as I have said, are wired inside-out, with the nerve fibers from the retina running into the interior of the globe. To reach the brain, the fibers have to dive through a hole at the back of the eye. There are no photoreceptors where the hole is, so there the retina is blind. This is why we have blind spots (and octopuses, whose eyes are wired more sensibly, presumably don't). In Fig. 10.2, if you close your right eye and stare with your left at the dot you should be able, by moving the book closer to your face or further away, to maneuver the black star onto your blind spot and make it disappear. Natural selection has arranged that the blind spots of our two eyes don't overlap, so normally we see no gaps in our visual fields when we have both eyes open.

Large foveae would also change our social behavior, as 'eye contact' would be far less specific. In the Counting Crows' song *Mr. Jones*, the line, 'she's looking at you . . . no she's looking at me' would become, 'we're all in her visual field'.

Noise

The word *noise* comes from the Latin *nausea*. In everyday English it means a disturbing sound, but in information theory it means contamination of any kind of signal.

If not for noise, a single neuron could carry infinite information. Its firing rate can vary smoothly between zero spikes per second and some maximum. So the number of possible different firing rates is technically infinite; for instance it might be 11 spikes per second or 11.1 or 11.11 and so on. Or maybe the number of possibilities isn't infinite (if time itself resolves into a finite sequence of moments at a quantum scale), but at least it is extremely large. Let us say it is infinite. How many yes-or-no questions do you need to specify one of an infinity of possibilities? Infinitely many questions. So by Shannon's criterion the information carried in the firing rate of a single noiseless neuron at any moment is infinitely many bits.

Fig. 10.2 The blind spot.

Now add noise. Suppose the neuron reports skin temperatures between 0 and 100 °C. The code is 1 spike per second for every degree, but noise causes random fluctuations of, say, plus or minus 1 spike per second. When the cell fires at 50 spikes per second, the real temperature might be anywhere between 49 and 51 °C. So noise introduces uncertainty and therefore lowers the information content of the message. Roughly speaking, you now know the temperature to an accuracy of only about 2 °C, so the range from 0 to 100 °C is divided into only about fifty bins. Fifty is somewhat less than two to the sixth power, so on average you need only six or fewer yes-or-no questions to distinguish fifty possibilities. Therefore the information content of the neuron's message is about 6 bits. The exact number of bits depends on several details, but in any case it is a steep drop from the infinite information carried by the noiseless neuron. In some ways the metaphor of 'contamination' doesn't do justice to the disruptive power of noise, where a small jitter in a signal can drastically reduce its information content.

Noisy sensors

Our sensors are designed for the efficient transfer of information. A simple example is the semicircular canals. D. A. Robinson pointed out that their design minimizes the effects of noise. On each side of the head are three canals. Each canal measures the component of head rotation in its own plane, and each canal plane lies at roughly right angles to the others. Figure 10.3A shows the advantage of the orthogonal arrangement. For simplicity only two canals are drawn, and they are represented abstractly as two orthogonal lines, one horizontal and one vertical, like the axes of a graph. The black dot between the axes is head velocity. It projects along the dashed lines onto the two canals. White dots on the axes represent these projections; they are the velocity components measured by the canals. Through each white dot runs a thick line representing noise: given the head velocity in the picture, the firing rate of the nerve fibers from the canals can vary over these ranges. To reconstruct the head velocity, the

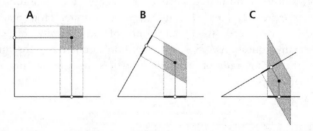

Fig. 10.3 The rhombus of doubt is smallest when the sensors lie at right angles to each other.

brain in effect runs the projections in reverse, along the dotted lines. Owing to noise, the reverse-projected reconstruction of head velocity may lie anywhere in the stippled square (or, more generally, given that it isn't a square any more when the canals aren't at right angles, let us call it a stippled rhombus). And conversely, given any reconstruction, the brain can't be sure that it matches the real head velocity, but it knows that the real velocity lies somewhere in the rhombus of uncertainty. The area of the rhombus is a measure of the brain's uncertainty about head velocity. Robinson pointed out that the rhombus is smallest when the two canals lie at right angles to one another. As the angle becomes more and more obtuse or acute, the rhombus grows larger and larger, becoming a little narrower but a lot longer, as shown in Figs. 10.3B and C. Its area is proportional to the cosecant of the angle between the canals, or in other words to one divided by the sine of the angle. It is smallest when the canals are orthogonal, and grows to infinity as the canals rotate toward parallel. This is probably the main reason that the three semicircular canals on each side of the head are close to orthogonal.

Noisy neurons

Internal messages within the brain also are contaminated with noise. Christopher Harris and Daniel Wolpert have shown that the form of this internal noise may explain some otherwise puzzling things about sensorimotor processing.[178] They argue that neural noise is signal dependent: the harder the neurons fire, the noisier they are, or in other words the more randomly variable their firing rates become. This pattern, they show, has implications throughout motor control.

For instance we have seen that saccadic eye movements are controlled in a way that optimizes speed and accuracy. Harris and Wolpert point out that the optimal neural commands for this task depend on the pattern of noise in the brain. They assume, as I did earlier, that the saccadic system is trying to minimize the difference between current and desired eye position, summed over time. The way to manage this, in the absence of noise, is to drive the eye as fast as possible to its goal because then you minimize the time when you are off target. But Harris and Wolpert point out that noise in the neural network tends to jostle the eye off its course. If the intensity of the noise were always the same, regardless of neural activity, then the best option would still be to drive the eye as fast as possible. But if neural noise is signal dependent—if it increases when the neurons fire harder—then you can reduce noise and make more accurate saccades by reducing neuron firing, though that means your saccades will be slower than they might have been because the neural commands driving them are weaker. So signal-dependent noise forces the brain to compromise between accuracy and speed. It is a matter of everyday experience that bodily movements are less accurate when they are faster.

In their simulations Harris and Wolpert chose a saccade target, and a duration for the saccade that was slightly longer than the minimum possible for their simulated control system, and they computed the neural command that would drive the eye to the target in the allotted time with the minimum variance, meaning that if you ran thousands of saccades with this profile, the average inaccuracy would be as small as possible. The resulting saccade, they found, matched the kinematics of real saccades. Presumably the brain's procedure differs slightly from Harris and Wolpert's: it probably doesn't choose a duration for its saccade arbitrarily and then make the most accurate movement compatible with that time frame. More likely speed and accuracy are balanced against one another, some combination of the two being optimized. But the results would be much the same.

Harris and Wolpert use signal-dependent noise to explain various features of arm control as well, for instance the speed-curvature law, which says that when you swing your arm in an arc, as for example when you spray-paint an ellipse on a wall, then the speed of your hand is proportional to the negative-one-third power of the local curvature of its path. That is, your hand moves faster along the straighter stretches, slower round tight curves.

For both eye and arm, the effects that Harris and Wolpert attribute to noise containment can also be explained in other ways. We get some of the same effects if we propose that the brain tries to reduce the firing rates of motor neurons, not as a way of quelling noise but simply to save fuel. But Harris and Wolpert make a convincing case that signal-dependent noise is an important factor in sensorimotor transformations.

They point out also that the optimal control patterns for coping with noise could be learned using simple error signals. In the case of saccades, it could be the same error signal that I suggested earlier for training a noiseless network, namely the difference between desired and actual eye position summed over time. Presented with this error signal, a noiseless adaptive network will learn to make the fastest saccades it can. Present the same error signal to a network loaded with signal-dependent noise, and the error signal will reflect the effects of that noise. The network will reduce its firing, Harris-and-Wolpert style, to make slightly slower, more accurate saccades.

Good and bad noise

I have been discussing how noise causes problems for the brain, but it may also play more useful roles. Sometimes noise can actually make a weak signal easier to decipher: if the signal itself is too tiny to discern, the superimposed noise may still now and then exceed the threshold of detection. From the pattern of detectable noise we may be able to deduce something about the subliminal signal. Noise may also allow the brain to create unpredictable behavior. If you watch a housefly's erratic cruising, it is easy to believe that it is using a noise generator to plot a course its enemies won't be able to predict. Our own brains may use noise in a similar way, to help generate creative thoughts.

Normally, though, noise hampers the flow of information through the brain. So natural selection has designed our sensors, effectors, and probably most of our internal wiring in a way that minimizes the disruption. And our adaptive networks can learn to cope with noise. Patterns of noise are reflected in the error signals that guide learning, so the noise itself can shape the brain, optimizing the way it handles information.

Chapter 11

Inference

Hermann von Helmholtz observed that sensory perception is a form of unconscious inference. Given a stream of signals from a variety of sensors, all of them noisy, all of them limited also in other ways, your brain has to infer what is going on in the outside world. Your sense organs routinely deliver incomplete, inaccurate, or contradictory reports. When you creep up the stairs to murder a sleeping houseguest, your eyes may report that there is a dagger floating in the air before you, the handle toward your hand, but your fingers, when you try to clutch it, may say that there isn't. Your senses are fooled by stereo equipment, by virtual reality, by drugs, and by optical illusions. Just turning down the lights makes your visual sense unreliable. You should think of the motor systems of the brain as a submarine crew, desperately trying to gain vital information from the dials and flickering screens of the vessel's battle-damaged sensors. My own submarine experience is limited to touring the set of *Das Boot*, so I am forced to explain the principles of sensory inference using a more prosaic analogy involving thermometers, but you can still imagine someone desperately trying to gain vital information from battle-damaged thermometers in a combat submarine.

Your lying senses

You are desperately trying to measure the temperature of something using two thermometers. Owing to design faults, neither thermometer is guaranteed always to deliver accurate readings, nor do the two thermometers usually agree with each other. In this way they are like two liars who haven't managed to coordinate their stories, but they are also like your senses. How do you make the best possible guess about the temperature given your untrustworthy instruments? First we need to understand what is meant by an unreliable sensor.

Distortion

Thinking of features you wouldn't want in a sensor, you may think first of distortion—you don't want the sensor to warp its signals—but in fact a consistent distortion is not a problem, at least not in the absence of noise. We would have no serious difficulty using a distorting thermometer, say one that at low temperatures registers each degree of warming with a 1 mm rise in its mercury but that at higher temperatures becomes less sensitive, registering each degree of warming with only a 0.5 mm rise. Reading this instrument naively would lead to errors, but if we know its quirks we can correct for them by redrawing the scale beside the mercury tube, crowding the tick marks closer together at the top of the range. In the brain, similarly, data from a distorting sense organ could be interpreted by correcting for the distortion.

But distortion isn't entirely irrelevant to sensor function, because of its interaction with noise. Distortion can make a detector relatively insensitive over part of its input range. In the presence of noise, this insensitivity can increase uncertainty. If the mercury level jitters over a 0.5 mm range when the temperature is constant, then we can trust our distorting thermometer to within 0.5 °C in its more sensitive, lower range, but only to within 1 °C in its less sensitive upper range. The uneven spread of uncertainty may be a problem, but it may also be useful if for some reason we need more accuracy in the lower range. So distortion can serve a purpose.

Variability

A more serious problem is noise itself, which causes a sensor to give different responses to identical stimuli. I will assume that it gives accurate readings on average, though any individual measurement is likely to be somewhat off (I will discuss this assumption later). With this sort of sensor, if you measure the temperature over and over again, say a thousand times, when it is in fact exactly 28 °C, then the average of all thousand readings will be about 28, and if you take a million readings the average will be even closer to 28, but the individual readings will vary. The more variable the sensor, the less reliable is any one of its readings.

Variability is quantified using what statisticians call the variance, which we compute by taking each reading, subtracting it from the average of all the readings, squaring the difference, adding up the squares, and dividing by the number of readings; if the readings are 27, 27, 28, and 30, then the average reading is 28 and the variance is $[(-1)^2 + (-1)^2 + 0^2 + 2^2]/4 = (1 + 1 + 0 + 4)/4 = 6/4 = 1.5$. The more the readings are scattered, the larger is their variance, and the less reliable is the sensor.

How can we interpret contradictory, unreliable signals? The Hungarian-born engineer Rudolf Kalman devised a method based on weighted averaging, giving more weight to the more trustworthy sensor, much as you might read a news story in two newspapers and give more credence to the paper that folds out big and less credence to the tabloid.[179] If the thermometers read 26 and 32 °C, and both are equally reliable, you average their reports to get an estimate of 29 °C. If the first thermometer, reading 26 °C, is twice as reliable as the other, you might give it twice as much weight, computing an estimate of two times 26 °C plus one times 32 °C, all divided by three, to yield 28 °C. Notice that this estimate is closer to the report given by the more reliable sensor.

Kalman's recipe for reading two thermometers is this. First learn their variances. Then when you want to interpret a pair of readings from the two, multiply each reading by the variance of the *other* thermometer, add the two products together, and divide by the sum of the variances. In other words, take a weighted average of the two readings, using as the weighting factor for each thermometer the variance of the other one. This weighting makes intuitive sense because it means that the more reliable thermometer, with the smaller variance, gets the larger weighting. If Kalman had three thermometers, he would weight each one by the product of the variances of the other two. If he had four or more unreliable thermometers, he would turn on the Weather Network. Kalman proved that, given certain reasonable assumptions, his formula yields the most accurate estimate of temperature, on average, that can be obtained from the readings. But there is more to Kalman's achievement than fiddling with cheap thermometers. He applied the same ideas to the more complex case where multiple sensors monitor dynamic processes, unfolding according to linear equations, and he discovered the optimal linear processor for interpreting the data. This processor, called the Kalman filter, is a crucial component in much of our technology.

Does the brain use Kalman filters to interpret its sensory inputs? Probably it shouldn't. For one thing, Kalman assumes that the variance of each sensor is always the same regardless of the value of the quantity being measured; that is, if you take a thousand readings when the temperature is 28 °C and you find that the thermometer's variance is 2, then when you use the same thermometer to take a thousand readings at 36 °C you will find the same variance. This assumption holds in many engineering applications but probably not for biological sensors and neurons. As I said in the last chapter, at least some neurons appear to carry signal-dependent noise, firing more variably when they encode more intense signals. This is one reason why Kalman's theory may not apply directly to the brain.

Kalman further assumed that when the temperature is constant at 28 °C, then repeated sensor readings will average exactly 28 °C. That may sound optimistic for biological sense organs, but all it means is that the brain has correctly calibrated its sensors. It has learned their quirks, learned to interpret their readings with no systematic error (though it will still make errors owing to noise). So this assumption of Kalman's is biologically plausible.

But the main strike against Kalman filters in the brain is that they are the best estimators only for *linear* systems. As most sensorimotor systems are highly nonlinear, the brain needs some more general form of inference that is not restricted to linearity. The most general approach to this question is what is called the Bayesian approach.

Optimal inference

Ultimately, sensory inference is a matter of conditional probabilities. The conditional probability of some event A, given some other event B, is the likelihood that A will occur if B occurs. The probability that the sidewalk is wet may be low in general, but the conditional probability that it is wet given that it is raining is high. When the brain interprets a sensory signal, it has to figure out the conditional probability, given that signal, that some state of affairs holds in the world (ultimately, of course, the brain uses its information about states of the world to shape motor performance—I will get to that later). Given that the vestibular sensors are firing in such and such a pattern, what is the likelihood that the head is rotating at 100 degrees per second rightward, or 90 degrees per second, or 110? What is the most likely head velocity, given that vestibular signal?

The brain favors likely interpretations, obviously, because they are more likely to be correct. It is uncomfortable with apparent flukes or coincidences. In Fig. 11.1A, for instance, the line drawing is seen as a cube, whereas in Fig. 11.1B it is not seen as a slightly rotated cube but as a flat arrangement of triangular tiles making a hexagon. Why does the perception change so markedly, even though both figures are equally consistent with a cube? Presumably because for a cube to look like Fig. 11.1B the front and rear corners would have to be perfectly aligned, and the brain considers this coincidence too unlikely and therefore rejects the interpretation. If the depicted shape were a flat pattern of tiles, no unlikely circumstances would be needed to explain the picture, and so that interpretation is accepted. This same wisdom underlies the principle of medical diagnosis, 'If you

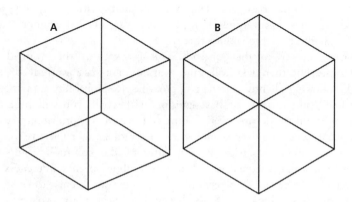

Fig. 11.1 The two drawings are similar, but the left one is seen as a cube and the right one as a flat pattern of triangles making a hexagon.

hear hoof beats, don't look for zebras' (in African medical schools they must say something different). But how can the brain infer the likely interpretations?

Meet the Bayesians

The correct theory of optimal inference is what is often called Bayesian theory. Confusingly, though, that adjective is used in different ways by different people. It doesn't help that avowedly Bayesian writings sometimes seem to be trying to promote an air of mystery or conspiracy. They speak of 'conversion' to Bayesianism, or thank some elder for 'helping me recognize that I am a Bayesian.' After a while, it starts to sound like a cult, or a society for mutual aid like the Freemasons. Who are these Bayesians, with their secret handshakes, their subterranean temples, their ridiculous robes and helmets? And what does it take to join?

The main entry requirement is that you embrace a certain interpretation of the concept of probability. As a home test for Bayesian nature, ask yourself this question: given a fair coin, what exactly does it mean to say that its probability of landing heads is one half? Is this just a compact way of saying that, if you threw the coin very many times, the number of heads would tend to be about a half of the total, and would draw closer and closer to one half as the number of throws approached infinity? If you believe that, you are a filthy 'Frequentist', an enemy of Bayesianism. Or do you believe that the one-half frequency of heads is not a definition of their one-half probability but a consequence of it? Do you think that probability is the same thing as plausibility, which is a basic, unanalyzable concept and which, like other ground-level concepts such as truth and falsity in logic, obeys a set of axioms or rules which must simply be accepted as part of the structure of the world? If you believe this, you have the right stuff to be a Bayesian. This was apparently the viewpoint of the Reverend Thomas Bayes himself and maybe also of Pierre-Simon Laplace, the main architect of probability theory.

A correct answer to that question will get you in the front door of Bayes House, but then you will find yourself in a dark warren of passageways, all following slightly different approaches to probability and inference, all in some sense variants of Bayesianism. In the halls you will hear a continuous murmur of debate over the precise nature of probability, whether and in what sense it is epistemological or ontological, subjective or objective, in the mind or outside it. But little of the controversy appears to have any practical consequences in terms of ruling specific inferences in or out. Even the Bayesians' objection to Frequentism seems to be mainly esthetic: they just think it is needlessly complicated to explain a basic concept like plausibility by invoking a hypothetical infinite string of coin tosses. They object especially when the issue is the probability of a non-repeatable event. Suppose the probability is 50 per cent that taking this

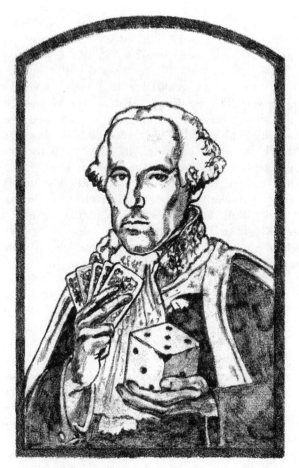

Fig. 11.2 Pierre-Simon Laplace, architect of probability and inference theory.

medicine now will cure me. To most Bayesians this means simply that the statement 'It will cure me' has a value halfway between pure truth and pure falsehood, whereas a Frequentist has to start spinning tales about how, if there were very many people like me, whose clinical conditions were identical to mine in all relevant respects as far as we can measure them, then about half of us would be cured by taking the medicine, and the more patients there were in total, the closer the cured fraction would come to one half. But it seems likely that computations by careful Frequentists will produce the same answers as Bayesian procedures, and will often look similar internally as well. There are other controversies that do have practical repercussions for inference, a major one being the issue of priors, which I will discuss in a moment. But as for the practical corner-stone of Bayesian inference, Bayes' rule, no one questions its validity.

Bayes' rule

Bayesian inference relies on Bayes' rule, which is a formula for computing conditional probabilities. It starts from the fact that if we know the probability of B, $P(B)$, and we know the conditional probability of A given B, $P(A|B)$, then we can find the probability of A and B both occurring, $P(A \& B)$, by multiplying: $P(A \& B) = P(A|B)P(B)$. For example, if the probability $P(B)$ that Betty will attend the party is 0.25, and the probability $P(A|B)$ that Archie will attend if Betty does is 0.8, then the probability $P(A \& B)$ that both Archie and Betty will show up is the product, $0.8 \times 0.25 = 0.2$. Obviously we can reverse the roles of A and B, so we have a second formula for the probability of A and B occurring, $P(A \& B) = P(B|A)P(A)$. Both formulae have to give the same result, so we know that $P(A|B)P(B) = P(B|A)P(A)$. Dividing both sides of this equation by $P(B)$, we get $P(A|B) = P(B|A)P(A)/P(B)$, which is Bayes' rule.

For sensorimotor applications, let us replace the letter B in this formula by the letter S, representing some pattern of activity in your sensors; and we will replace A by E, representing some event in the world. I will assume that the brain knows the probabilities of S and E, $P(S)$ and $P(E)$. In other words, it has a good idea what percentage of the time the sensors are firing in pattern S and it knows what percentage of the time E is the case.[180] This knowledge may have been learned or it may be innate, but in any case it is available. I will assume also that the brain knows the statistical properties of its own sense organs; in particular, it knows the conditional probability that the sensor will show activity pattern S if event E occurs, $P(S|E)$. With this information and Bayes' rule, the brain can compute the more useful quantity $P(E|S)$, the conditional probability that event E is occurring, given that the sensor activity is S.

You think you see your Uncle Elmer, but it is dark outside so the probability that you would have this sensory impression if he were really there is only 50 per cent, $P(S|E) = 0.5$. Elmer lives on this street, and the chances that he would be out walking here at this hour are 10 per cent, $P(E) = 0.1$. When you are strolling here at night, you quite often think you see Uncle Elmer; sometimes he is there and sometimes he isn't, but 20 per cent of the time you have the sensory impression, so $P(S) = 0.2$. How likely is it that Elmer is really there, given that you seem to see him? By Bayes' rule it is $P(E|S) = P(S|E)P(E)/P(S) = 0.5 \times 0.1/0.2 = 0.25$—the chances are just one in four that Elmer is there. And how likely is it that your brain would really contain these quantitative estimates of probabilities? It is very unlikely that they would be stored in such a way that you could verbalize them, but I will argue later that it is plausible that your neural networks could learn to behave as if they were using Bayes' rule with roughly suitable probabilities. And of course the idea is not that you consciously calculate through the options. Rather your perceptual networks do the math behind the veil of consciousness and deliver a verdict, or suggestion, which you experience as the conviction, or inkling, that Uncle Elmer is around.

Priors

Of all the factors in Bayes' formula, the one that is hardest to estimate is often $P(E)$, which is called the prior probability of the event E. It is called the prior probability to distinguish it from the posterior, or conditional, probability of E after the sense data arrive, which is $P(E|S)$. Prior probabilities may be hard to estimate, but they are important. If you know that Uncle Elmer is dead, then $P(E)$ is zero, and so, by Bayes' rule, is the probability that you have spotted him out walking, whatever your sensors may tell you. In the medical maxim, it is the prior improbability of zebras that makes them an unlikely guess when you hear hoof beats.

Often in practice, we simply have no information at all about prior probabilities. In that case, our task is to infer in a way that admits our ignorance, that doesn't accidentally assume any knowledge we don't really have. As it turns out, this is a subtle and difficult matter, and a topic of intensive research. To get a sense of the problem, consider the simplest case: you are told that one of two events, A or B, is going to happen. You know that exactly one of them will occur. The possibility that both or neither might come to pass is entirely ruled out. But that is all you know. About the probabilities of A and B you are told nothing. You have no background data to shape any estimate. This situation arises often enough in real life. If you need those probabilities to serve as the priors for some calculation, what should you do?

Bayesian policy is to apply the principle of indifference, which says that A and B should be assumed to be equally likely, so each has probability 0.5. This rule is old (it goes back at least to the great seventeenth-century Swiss mathematician Jacob Bernoulli) and to many people it sounds sensible: if you have no reason to regard one event as more likely than the other, the fair thing is to assume that they are equally probable. To other people, though, that assumption seems every bit as arbitrary as any other. The Bayesian viewpoint is this: we are trying to formulate a procedure for deducing probabilities. Certainly, one requirement of any valid procedure is that our calculations should depend only on the facts we have, and not on how the facts are named or labeled. So if our recipe told us to assign a probability of 0.8 to A and 0.2 to B then two statisticians, presented with the same data but with the labels A and B switched, would arrive at different conclusions. The only way to make our deductions independent of arbitrary labeling is to adopt the principle of indifference, which assigns A and B equal probabilities of 0.5.

But there can be problems applying the principle. Suppose you learn that a variable, x, lies in the range 0 to 10. Being otherwise ignorant of x, you apply the principle of indifference. For instance, one-tenth of the range of possible values for x lies between 1 and 2, so you assume that x lies between 1 and 2 with probability 1/10, or 0.1. By identical reasoning, x lies between 8 and 9 with the same probability. Now suppose that later, for another calculation, you need the prior probabilities for a related variable y, which is equal to x^2. Of course you know that y lies between 0^2 and 10^2, that is, between 0 and 100, but what are the probabilities within that range? If you stand by your earlier guess about the probabilities of x, then you have to conclude that y has a 0.1 chance of lying between 1 and 4 (that is between 1^2 and 2^2), and the same chance of lying between 64 and 81 (8^2 and 9^2). But if you forget your earlier guess about x and apply the principle of indifference directly to y, you get a different answer, where y lies between 1 and 4 with a probability of just $(4-1)/100$, or 0.03, and between 64 and 81 with a probability of $(81-64)/100$, or 0.17. Of course this result logically implies that x lies between 1 and 2 with probability 0.03 and between 8 and 9 with probability 0.17, clashing badly with your original guesses of 0.1 for both. You are mired in contradictions. Statisticians have devised some principles for coping with issues like these, but the question isn't entirely settled. For many sensorimotor systems, though, I will suggest later that the problem is solved by natural selection, via hard-wiring and learning. For these systems, the bottom line is sensorimotor performance, and an adaptive network will automatically learn whatever set of priors optimizes its performance.

Minimizing error

With Bayes' rule you—meaning your unconscious inferential machinery—can compute the alternative probabilities that what you see is Uncle Elmer or Uncle Oscar or Elvis Presley or the Sasquatch or whatever. Knowing all this, your brain can make the most reasonable guess as to what is out there being sensed. But what is the most reasonable guess? One option is to choose the most likely situation in the world, given the sensory activity. If Uncle Oscar comes out with the highest conditional probability, choose him.

But it is often a better strategy to choose not the interpretation that is most likely but the one that will be closest to correct on average. For instance, suppose that a given pattern of sensor activity means 34 per cent of the time that some variable has value 0, 33 per cent of the time that it has value 1, and the remaining 33 per cent of the time that it has value 2. Then the likeliest value is 0, but if you choose that interpretation you will sometimes be wrong by as much as 2 units, and on average you will be 0.99 units away from the correct value. If instead you guess that the value is 1, you will never be in error by more than 1 unit, and your average error will be just 0.67. This strategy, which is called minimizing expected error, can make both your average and maximum errors smaller than they would be if you chose the most likely interpretation.

Your errors should be measured by their impact on your genetic success. Some perceptual errors are costlier than others. It is worse to mistake your boss for a punching bag than the other way round. You are better off chatting politely with a punching bag than battering the president.

A simple example comes up in the VOR: if horizontal eye velocity is inaccurate—if it doesn't exactly balance horizontal head velocity—then images will slide across your fovea, impairing your vision. But equal-sized errors in torsional eye velocity—in the eye's spin about its own line of sight—may not be so serious as they merely make the visual world spin around the fovea; the center of the foveal image itself, like the pole star, is stationary and clear. So horizontal errors matter more than torsional errors. As we would expect, there is evidence that the error signals that shape the VOR reflect the primacy of the fovea.

Bayes in the colliculus

Thomas Anastasio and colleagues have found signs of Bayesian inference in the superior colliculus, which is a center for space perception, located in the roof of the midbrain.[181] Its cells receive sensory signals of various kinds, conveying sight, hearing, touch, and the sense of body position. This is one of the few places in the brain to receive signals directly from the retina. In reptiles and amphibians it is called the optic tectum, and it is the closest thing they have to our visual cortex. In humans the superior colliculus may play a role in blindsight—the rudimentary visual abilities, detectable only with specialized tests, of people who otherwise appear to be completely blind owing to cortical damage. But the colliculus is multisensory, not just visual; in parts of it over half of the neurons are multimodal—they respond to more than one sensory modality, say sight and sound or sight and touch.

Anastasio suggests that the activity of collicular cells reflects their conviction that a target is present—their firing rates code the conditional probabilities that a target lies in the cell's receptive field, given the sensory signals reaching the cell. With this hypothesis, Anastasio can explain much of the cells' behavior. For instance, a typical multimodal neuron responds more vigorously to combined stimulation, a sight and a sound, than to either stimulus alone. The combined response is not just the sum of the individual responses. It may be ten times stronger than the reaction to either modality alone. This is called multisensory enhancement. A similar effect is seen in the orienting behavior of whole animals. A light and a sound occurring at the same time and in the same place can prompt an animal to turn toward them even when the individual stimuli, presented alone, are too weak. From a Bayesian viewpoint, this is understandable. When two modalities report the same thing, its conditional probability rises. Anastasio shows that the quantitative behavior of the cells is consistent with a Bayesian computation of conditional probability.

Multisensory enhancement is usually strongest when the individual stimuli are weak, and dwindles as they strengthen. When the individual stimuli are powerful, multisensory enhancement is gone: the response to combined stimuli is scarcely stronger than the response to either one alone, and much weaker than the sum of the single responses. This feature is called inverse effectiveness. It may simply reflect saturation, but it is also predicted by Bayes' rule, and it is perfectly intuitive as an inferential mechanism: if an individual signal is strong and clear, you may be certain of your interpretation based on it alone, so a second signal does nothing to strengthen your conviction. Only when a signal is weak and ambiguous can you boost your confidence by receiving a second signal. If you see a friend directly before you on a clear, sunny day, the sight alone will be enough to convince you of their presence. The familiar sound of their voice won't make much difference to your certainty.

On the other hand, imagine that you are sitting with your eyes shut and you hear your friend's voice directly ahead of you. You are fairly sure that they are present, but when you open your eyes you see no sign of them anywhere, no visible body to go with the voice. Now you are less certain, because your senses are in conflict. This is why, according to Anastasio, bimodal collicular cells fire less than unimodal ones in the presence of only one sensory modality. The bimodal cells are confused by the missing modality, while the unimodal cells notice nothing amiss.

Vestibular inference

A well-studied case of neural inference involves the vestibular system, which has to deduce from its sensor readings the head's translational motion and its tilt relative to gravity. It needs to distinguish these two things, motion and tilt, to run a number of reflexes: the VOR that holds your gaze line stable in space, and various postural reflexes that keep you upright. The slight hitch here is that it is physically impossible to distinguish these variables, according to Albert Einstein's principle of equivalence.

The principle of equivalence

Imagine yourself standing in a closed capsule. Your feet are pressed against the floor. When you let go of things they fall down. To all appearances, you are standing in a gravitational force field, as in daily life on Earth, but is there another possibility? This is the question that led Einstein to his famous principle of equivalence and from there to general relativity and the overthrow of Newtonian physics.

Einstein said, maybe you aren't on Earth. Maybe you are outside any significant gravitational field, flying through empty space in your capsule, with rocket engines accelerating the capsule upward; that is, in the direction away from your feet and toward your head. Not gravity but rather acceleration is pressing your feet against the floor, just as it presses your back against the seat when your car accelerates. Released objects seem to fall toward the floor because the capsule is accelerating upward around them. Einstein conjectured that it is impossible, by any experiment whatever, for you in your capsule to determine whether you are accelerating or sitting stationary in a gravitational field. In fact, there is no distinction between gravitation and acceleration—this is the principle of equivalence. From it, Einstein deduced a set of bizarre consequences which have since been verified experimentally with great precision, for example the bending of light rays and the slowing of time near massive objects. So the principle is considered well supported.

It is often said that the human vestibular organs are in the same predicament as Einstein's space traveler. Sitting inside the labyrinth, they are trying to detect the direction of gravity and also the acceleration of the head. The detectors are the otolith organs, utricle and saccule. They are sheets of jelly, one horizontal and one vertical sheet on each side of the head, each embedded with many dense crystals called otoliths. Nerve cells detect the motions of the otoliths in their jelly matrix. If you tilt your head clockwise, your otoliths hang down toward your right ear. If you accelerate leftward, your otoliths are flung toward your right ear. Thanks to the equivalence principle, the otolith motions are the same whether they are caused by tilt or acceleration, so how does the brain distinguish? (Other organs besides the otoliths may sense gravity and acceleration—the kidneys swaying on their stalks are candidates—but this doesn't change the problem.)

One difference between your vestibular system and Einstein's space traveler is that you are not trying to distinguish acceleration from gravitation in any absolute sense. You are trying to estimate your acceleration relative to your surroundings: relative to the Earth, usually, or to the interior of a train carriage or airplane cabin or space capsule. There would be no point trying to distinguish absolute acceleration from gravitation; as Einstein said, there *is* no distinction, so there are no sensorimotor consequences. But there *is* a point to detecting relative acceleration. If your otoliths are flung toward your right ear because you are accelerating leftward relative to your surroundings, then you should respond by accelerating your eyes rightward, to keep the images of those surroundings stable on your retinas. But if your otoliths are hanging toward your right ear because your head is tilted clockwise, or right-ear down, then rightward eye motion would be pointless; you might be better off rolling your eyes counterclockwise, to keep them better aligned with the horizon. So relative acceleration and tilt have sensorimotor implications.

Relative tilt and acceleration can be sensed visually and sometimes by hearing and touch. But when the lights go out, you often need to estimate them using the otolith organs alone, which can't see or hear or feel your surroundings. All you have to go on is the ambiguous shifting of your otoliths. So in the dark, the vestibular system is in a worse predicament than Einstein's space traveler. It has ambiguous data but a real decision to make, about tilt and acceleration relative to the unseen surroundings. Not surprisingly, it doesn't work perfectly. Sometimes you do confuse tilt and motion. But usually you can distinguish them. How do you manage it?

Prior improbabilities

You exploit prior knowledge. Imagine yourself back in Einstein's thought experiment, or in this slight variant of it: you wake up in your own bedroom with the curtains closed, so that your view of the outside world is blocked. You want to know your acceleration relative to the Earth. On a typical morning, how many experiments do you do before deciding whether your bedroom is sitting still in the Earth's gravitational field or rocketing through space?

From a lifetime of experience you know that the rocket scenario is implausible. Every time you lie on your back in bed, your otoliths register a constant gravitational force of $9.8 \, N \, kg^{-1}$ toward the back of your head. According to Einstein, this force is indistinguishable from a forward acceleration, in the direction of your nose, of $9.8 \, m \, s^{-2}$. If you lay on your back for 1 min, that noseward acceleration would bring you to a speed of about $589 \, m \, s^{-1}$, or $2119 \, km \, h^{-1}$. If you interpreted your otolith activity this way, you would have to conclude that, over this 1 min, you had moved 17.7 km from your starting point along a straight line, putting you in the middle stratosphere, entering the ozone layer. In about 2.5 h, you would cross the moon's orbit and you would be moving at $88 \, km \, s^{-1}$ (disappointingly, it would take nearly a day and a half to get to Mars this way, even if you went to bed during an optimal launch window, and you would need almost a year to reach light speed).[182] On this interpretation of your sense data, the proper motor response is to flail around, dodging asteroids in that realm where no one can hear you scream. But your unconscious inferential machinery considers this interpretation less plausible than the correct one, that you are lying still in bed. Your vestibular system is not as open-minded as the passenger in Einstein's capsule.

For one thing, it knows that there is a gravitational field. It knows that the field is constant in time and uniform in space, always and everywhere pointing down, with a strength of 1g. Given any shift of the otoliths, the brain knows that part of the shift is caused by a gravitational pull of 1g, and the rest must reflect head acceleration. These assumptions serve us well, except on spacecraft in microgravity, where they may cause space sickness.

Knowing the strength of the field removes some of the ambiguity from the sensor readings, but not all of it. It suffices to rule out the space-flight interpretation when you are lying in bed—you sense a total acceleration of 1g, so if you think you are on your back, you have to attribute that whole acceleration to gravity, leaving no remainder for space travel. But you could still believe that your bed was upside down and you were accelerating at 2g, or $19.6 \, m \, s^{-2}$, toward the center of the Earth. Various oblique trajectories are also consistent with the otolith signal. These interpretations are all implausible, but how does the brain exclude them? It is not enough to say that they are silly. There must be some criterion, some mechanism by which the inferential networks avoid these interpretations when they compute head tilt and acceleration.

Temporal patterns

Gary Paige and others have suggested that the key to distinguishing tilt from acceleration is temporal pattern.[183, 184] Tilt is often sustained, whereas head accelerations are brief and changeable (if they weren't, they would fling our heads into the stratosphere). So if your otoliths are deviated toward your right ear by a constant force for several seconds or minutes, it is more likely that you are tilted sideways, lying on your right ear, than that you are undergoing a sustained, constant leftward acceleration. Paige proposed that the brain puts the otolith signals through temporal filters. A high-pass filter screens out the relatively constant otolith signals evoked by tilt relative to gravity, so everything that passes through is fairly likely to reflect head acceleration. A low-pass filter similarly screens out the high-frequency jitter of head acceleration, passing a fairly pure tilt signal to downstream processors.

This method is not completely reliable. So if Paige is correct, it should be possible to fool the vestibular sense, given the right stimuli. One way to experience these stimuli is to take one of those whirling bucket rides at a fairground. You stand with a group of people in the huge bucket, your backs to the cylindrical wall. The bucket starts to spin, faster and faster, and then the floor drops away, leaving you and the other paying customers stuck to the vertical wall by centrifugal force. What the otoliths feel, spinning inside the bucket, is a constant backward pull. They sense the sum of the centrifugal force and gravity, so the net force they register is an oblique one in the body's midline plane. The force is sustained and constant, so according to Paige, the brain should misinterpret it, as tilt rather than acceleration. Spun around in the laboratory version of the fairground bucket, subjects do tend to misperceive their motion as Paige predicts.[183] They misinterpret sustained, oblique forces as gravity, so they believe they are tipped relative to Earth-vertical.

Multisensory inference

I have repeatedly urged that optimization ideas are our best guide to the brain. Applying them now, it is clear that if the inferential engines of the vestibular sense are even close to optimal, they won't rely on temporal patterns alone to distinguish acceleration from tilt, but will use other sources of information. Theoretically there are other sources, and there is evidence that we use them. The vestibular sense is smarter than Paige's filters alone can explain.

Dora Angelaki and colleagues have shown that monkeys can distinguish tilts from accelerations even when they have the same temporal patterns.[185, 186] The monkeys oscillated sideways, back and forth on a sled track, or they rocked torsionally, tilting right-ear down and left-ear down at the same rate. Otolith inputs were nearly identical during the 2 motions, but even in darkness the monkeys could tell the difference: they always made appropriate eye movements, looking right and left when they slid sideways, counterrolling their eyes about the sight line when they tilted clockwise and counterclockwise. So the monkeys' brains use some clue besides temporal patterns to distinguish tilt from acceleration.

They do it by cross-matching signals from different sensors. Their (presumably) unconscious inference seems to run like this: 'My otolith organs are acting in a way that could mean either changing tilt or sideways acceleration. If I am tilting, then my rotation sensors—my semicircular canals—will detect the tilt. So if my canals report a tilt, I will choose that interpretation; otherwise, I must be accelerating sideways'. (I will discuss shortly how this sort of internal monolog can take place in a neural network.) As you would expect, inactivating the monkeys' semicircular canals erases their ability to distinguish the two stimuli in this experiment.

Multisensory cooperation can also work the other way—the otoliths can help the canals with their job of reporting head rotation. When you rotate about any axis except the Earth-vertical one, the rotation changes the direction of gravity relative to your head. If you do a somersault, the arrow of gravity rotates, circling in the midline plane. If you do a cartwheel, it circles in the frontal plane. The otolith sheets monitor the changing direction of gravity, providing the brain with another source of data on how the head is rotating. But this works only for rotations that are not about an Earth-vertical axis, because vertical-axis rotations don't change the direction of gravity relative to the head. For this reason, responses differ to turns about vertical and non-vertical axes. If you are spun in the dark at a constant rate about an Earth-vertical axis, like a merry-go-round, then your sense of movement lasts only about 40 seconds—as I have said earlier, the semicircular canals are high-pass filters so their response dies out after about 20 seconds of constant-speed spin, though the velocity-storage mechanism in the brain prolongs the sensation roughly twofold. But if you instead spin about an Earth-horizontal axis like a chicken on a barbecue spit, your sense of motion declines briefly at first but then holds steady for ever. Your canals soon fall silent, but your otolith organs continue to report the revolution of the gravity vector.

In theory there is another way that otoliths might detect head rotation. You have two sets of otolith organs on opposite sides of your head. During most rotations, the otoliths on the two sides are flung in different directions by the centrifugal force, like fairground riders on opposite sides of the spinning bucket. If you spin horizontally, the otoliths on your right side are flung to your right, those on your left side are flung to your left. Theoretically the brain could use these force differences to help compute the spin of the head, but apparently they are too small, during normal head movements, to be measured reliably amidst sensor noise, so this source of information is unavailable.

Other senses like vision, hearing, and touch can also help the brain estimate the body's motion. Vision can't monitor fast-changing head movements

because it is too slow, but for more leisurely motions vision becomes more important. You can verify this in a vivid way by going for an illusory ride in the Tumbling Room built by Ian Howard at York University in Toronto. Dr Howard leads you to a chair in a small kitchen, with stiff drapes on the windows and teacups glued to the table. Your chair is attached by a beam to the outside world, so that you stay upright while the kitchen slowly somersaults around you. But you feel that you are doing the turning. Midway through the somersault, you have a powerful impression that you are hanging upside down, even though your non-visual sensors all demur. Your otoliths say you are upright, your canals say you haven't moved, and, subjectively the most incongruous note, sensors in your backside indicate that you are still pressed against the chair seat. So the testimony of your eyes, combined with the prior knowledge that somersaulting rooms are unlikely, is enough to overcome the vestibular and tactile evidence that you are sitting upright. Vision is compelling, at least in a visual species like ours; moles or bats might be more impressed by revolving smells or echoes.

We probably use other, motor and cognitive, sources of information as well in inferring our own motion. Head motion, for instance, is often self-caused, so it should usually agree with sense data regarding neck and limb movement, and with our motor intentions. Maybe our vestibular sense can also use an internal representation of the surroundings and of the laws of physics, so that it mistrusts interpretations that would have us hovering in mid-air, burrowing through the ground, or walking through walls.

Networks of inference

How can the brain piece together all these data into an estimate of body motion? How can a neural network say to itself, 'My cupulas aren't deformed, so I must not be rotating'? There is no real puzzle here: it is just another computation. Some neurons in the network receive signals from the canals and otolith organs, and from the eyes, ears, and other sensors, coding a mix of data about motion and gravity. Other neurons drive the eye muscles. The point is to compute the optimal, compensatory eye movement, which among other things means coping with sensor noise, resolving ambiguity, performing something close to an optimal, Bayesian analysis of the available evidence.

Direct application of Bayesian formulae can be complex. It takes a lot of memory and processing capacity to store and manipulate the relevant probability distributions. But Bayesian inference can often be approximated by simple adaptive networks. All the network needs is an error signal that reflects its performance—a sensible error signal that reflects the catastrophic potential of various sorts of mistake, so that the network learns to chat with the punching bag rather than clobber the boss. Driven by this error signal, an adaptive network will adjust its synapses by the usual means until its average error is minimized. It is plausible, then, that our unconscious

inference is close to the Bayesian optimal, but that the standard equations of Bayesian inference are mirrored only abstractly in our brains. Neural networks may learn to infer with much less overhead and yet be roughly Bayesian in overall performance.

In the case of the VOR, models have been devised that perform part of this inference, computing head motion from canal and otolith signals, though for simplicity present theories still exclude vision, hearing, and other senses, and they assume noiseless signals. Two similar models have been developed, largely independently, by Stefan Glasauer and Dan Merfeld and their colleagues.[187, 188] In both models the computations are iterative. Signals coding the evolving estimates of head motion and position circulate repeatedly through the network, gradually settling to a final decision. In both models the network computes the inconsistency between the current estimates and the various sensor readings. For instance, if the otolith signals suggest a changing head tilt, and the current estimate of head motion reflects that idea, but the canals detect no such rotation, then there is an inconsistency. The network runs until it finds an estimate that makes all the discrepancies as small as possible. This is an optimization problem, and a nonlinear one, which means that its only known methods of solution are iterative. That is why both Glasauer and Merfeld posited looping neural circuits for the job, though as I have said earlier *our* inability to do a given job without iteration doesn't necessarily mean that the brain couldn't find a non-iterative method. A non-iterative procedure might run faster, as it wouldn't have to wait for the network to settle to a final decision.

Both the models and real brains make similar mistakes, misestimating head movement and posture in certain circumstances, for instance in the fairground bucket ride. But the reasons for error are probably different in models and reality. Glausauer and Merfeld's networks malfunction because their makers deliberately chose suboptimal values for some of their synapses, to make them act more like real monkeys and humans. In theory, the networks could be built to perform flawlessly. All you would have to do is this: to the canal signals, you apply perfect velocity storage; that is, you precisely undo the temporal filtering imposed by the sensors—this is mathematically possible, because the canal operator in the models is invertible. The result is a perfect estimate of head velocity. Use this to update your estimate of the direction of gravity relative to the head, yielding an equally perfect estimate of head tilt. Knowing the tilt, you can disambiguate the otolith signals to find translational acceleration.

In real life this can't work because noise interferes at every step. When the canals introduce unpredictable noise there is no way to remove it, to recover the true head velocity. And noisy neurons make it risky or impossible to build exactly the temporal operators you need for perfect estimation; for instance you can't build perfect integrators because they may explode. If we incorporate noise into future models of vestibular

inference, we may not have to introduce imperfections to make the models look more realistic. We may find that real errors are the result of optimal inference in the face of noise.

Glasauer and Merfeld's models don't learn multisensory inference; they have it built in from birth. But there is no obstacle to an adaptive model of the process. An adaptive network, driven by an appropriate error signal, in this case a signal coding retinal slip, could learn, by the mechanisms I have described in earlier chapters, to cope optimally with flawed sensors and internal noise. As usual, learning and hard-wiring are both viable methods of optimization. Optimal inference, like optimal dynamics, interfacing, iteration, and multidimensional control, can arise automatically as natural selection optimizes the sensorimotor performance of the brain.

Chapter 12

The search for intelligent life in the brain

I have argued for a threefold path through the functional interior of the brain: study sensorimotor systems, leave the details to computers, and identify the optimization principles that shaped performance. This approach yields insight and surprising, correct predictions about brain systems that might otherwise defy understanding. It applies equally to reflexive and cognitive functions: self-optimizing networks can learn and remember, they can recognize and create subtle patterns including temporal ones, they can predict the future and plan ahead, they can discern patterns hidden in noise, they can juggle probabilities and infer likely conclusions from data, they can engage in internal monologs about whether the head is really tilted, given that the otolith organs are signaling but the semicircular canals have reported no rotation. I have illustrated these ideas with relatively simple brain systems, but there is no reason why the method should stop working when it is applied to more complex ones. There is a continuum of neural systems stretching from primeval reflexes to the highest reaches of abstract thought. Our brains were built up by natural selection, starting from no brain at all, in tiny gradations. So it is reasonable to hope that we can proceed the same way, gradually increasing the scope and complexity of our simulations. How far we can go isn't yet clear, but at least there is little danger of any sudden roadblock halting our progress.

Unbroken line

Why does evolution proceed by tiny gradations? It is an optimizing process that drives its lineages down the slopes of an energy landscape, into basins of optimal fitness. It moves by genetic mutations and recombinations, retaining the ones that improve fitness, discarding the rest. The fitness-enhancing changes are overwhelming likely to be small changes.

What is wrong with large changes? A large, random alteration to any finely tuned machine is likely to be disastrous. If natural selection has brought you fairly close to a deep optimum, then your chances of landing even deeper by taking a flying leap into the unknown are negligible. Optimization algorithms built on this principle are uselessly slow even on the fastest computers. And remember that if you did manage to leap to a distant region of genetic space full of superhuman beings, superintelligent, strong, swift, and so on, you would still need at least one other reasonably agreeable mutant of the opposite sex to leap with you, landing genetically close enough to be your mate and give you children, or you wouldn't contribute much to evolution. Or maybe you don't need children: I can imagine a story where a sterile, superintelligent mutant of *Homo habilis* gives humanity a crucial push forward, say by inventing the wheel, and then perishes childless, but still the odds are against it. Chances are, we evolved by cumulative small changes in the genome.

Of course a small genetic change may make a big conceptual difference: a tiny genetic flaw can kill its bearer in childhood. And if a single base pair can mean the difference between life and death, couldn't it also, conceivably, mean the difference between consciousness and unconsciousness, or between intelligence and stupidity? Many people like this idea. They feel that, somewhere in human evolution, 'something happened': some small, fateful genetic change put us through a sort of phase transition, just as a tiny drop in temperature can transform liquid water into something completely different. That change vaulted us far beyond the other apes. I am not aware of any evidence for this idea, but certainly it is possible that, in this sense, our evolution included large leaps.

So we may have to make some conceptual leaps as we expand our brain simulations. But that will be true whether or not there was a phase transition in humanity's past. As I argued in Chapter 9, with the examples of non-commutativity, redundancy, and synergy, we have to expect new issues and concepts to emerge as we proceed, but we can still expect optimization ideas to guide us. We may need a little ingenuity to help us along, but I don't expect any conceptual barriers to force us from the three-fold path.

The bounds of computation

A greater danger is that we may gradually become overwhelmed as we take on more and more complex systems. Complexity is the main challenge for any approach to the brain, but at least the threefold path takes that challenge seriously and tries to deal with it. I have suggested that as we consider systems of higher and higher dimensions we can reasonably expect that the underlying optimization principles will proliferate only slowly. For instance eye–head coordination, which juggles at least fifteen degrees of freedom, can be understood based on a handful of optimized variables. The brain could learn to optimize these variables based on a handful of error signals carried by feedback loops. Simple feedback loops, acting in a complex environment, can yield arbitrarily complex behavior, so it is mathematically plausible that all our sensorimotor processing can be traced back to a relatively small number of fundamental loops. It is hard to guess the number, but I have argued that the brain is highly ordered and therefore simplifiable, and that the principles underlying the function of the entire brain may be remarkably few, given that natural selection has managed to zip its program for building brains into a single egg cell.

Granted, the program in the egg specifies only a protobrain: an organ that develops into a mature brain given appropriate input from the environment. Drawing out the implications of a brain-building program in a computer will be a complex task. To simulate the operation of a mature brain, we will need a computer with far more storage space than is required for the protobrain program itself. To simulate how the brain arises from the protobrain, driven by sensory signals from the external world, we will also need a good simulation of that world, or we will have to put the program into a robot that can sense and move in the real world. For large brain systems, the task may exceed our computer power and our patience. But so far, sensorimotor simulations have not approached either the limits of our computers or the complexity of the simulations used in astrophysics and meteorology. Future advances in computer technology will push the boundaries further outward, improving our prospects of simulating the sensorimotor performance of large subsystems of the human brain.

Thinking inside the box

Many neuroscientists want to look beneath performance and optimization principles at the underlying neural mechanisms. In some sense they want to decipher the contributions of the brain's component parts, say its neurons or nuclei. This is a vaguer, more difficult task and one whose feasibility and meaning I have questioned in this book, but I expect that with time its aims will be clarified and achieved to some extent. My point is merely that the prior goal of explaining sensorimotor performance is far more achievable and at least as interesting.

I would be thrilled to get my hands on a complete optimization profile of the human brain, say a computer simulation of the sensorimotor performance typical of healthy babies. Some scientists would say that even a complete sensorimotor description like the one I am imagining would still leave the brain a 'black box'. But these critics are underestimating the transparency of black boxes. If we have a full description of the adaptive performance of a machine, if we know what it will do in any more or less normal situation, then we know a great deal about it. It is true—and this is the chief complaint about black boxes—that even a complete input–output description is compatible with many different internal mechanisms, so it doesn't uniquely determine which mechanism is really at work. But compared with the range of mechanisms that were candidates before the input–output description was obtained, it narrows the field tremendously.

If you can specify the brain's adaptive performance, you rule out all but a minuscule fraction of its possible internal structures. So understanding the brain's performance is an extremely useful first step in working out its mechanisms. It is probably also a necessary step, because it is hard to deduce the mechanism by which an organ performs some function without knowing what that function is. And even if the internal mechanisms remain for ever inscrutable, the sensorimotor profile is valuable in its own right.

Sensorimotor mysteries

A sensorimotor approach may also clarify the supposed mysteries of neuro-science—the notions of consciousness, personal identity, knowledge, and representation. By representation I mean the connection between thoughts or wishes and the world. If I think that the chicken crossed the road to get to the other side, my thought is a pattern of brain activity, but it has some poorly understood connection with real chickens. If I want to go out this evening, my wish is another pattern of brain activity with some connection to events that may or may not happen in the future. So the fourth mystery is, what does it mean for a brain to believe or desire some state of affairs?

All four mysteries have occupied philosophers for millennia without yielding up complete solutions, but that doesn't mean that they are insoluble. Age-old questions may eventually succumb to reason, often in surprising ways and often as they pass from philosophy to science or mathematics (though the borders between the disciplines are hazy). That is what happened to old mysteries about the nature of space and time in the hands of Einstein, and to many ancient puzzles about infinity in the work of Georg Cantor. So it is plausible that the questions of consciousness, identity, knowledge, and representation may be swallowed up by science. In this case, the relevant branch of science is senso-rimotor biology.

Many questions about knowledge, for instance, may find answers within the developing theory of inference. That theory is full of controversy, as we saw in Chapter 11, but the prospects for consensus seem good if we focus on practical questions about statistical methodology; other differences, without practical consequences, can probably be accepted as alternative formulations of equivalent doctrines. The American physicist E. T. Jaynes took a step in that direction in his unfinished magnum opus, *Probability Theory: The Logic of Science*[189]. Jaynes stressed practical consequences, and based the whole subject of inference on a hypothetical robot that collects data and draws conclusions. The task of probability theory, as Jaynes saw it, is to work out how to program the robot so that it makes optimal use of its data. I think the next step is to empha-size that the optimal program for a robot depends on the details of its sensors and effectors, its environment, and its own aims or desires.

Optimal inference then passes into the territory of sensorimotor theory, and draws with it the issues of representation—belief and desire. Understanding identity, knowledge, and representation may take some time, but it helps to recognize what kind of issues these are: they are all sensorimotor questions.

Glossary

Algorithm. A procedure or set of rules for calculation or problem solving. Algorithms can be implemented by physical systems including computer programs and neural networks.

Algorithmic information content. Of a string of 0s and 1s: the shortest computer program (in a standardized computer language) that will cause the string to be printed out (by a standardized computer). Algorithmic information content is one measure of complexity.

Back-propagation. A learning mechanism for neural networks which strengthens or weakens the connections between the neurons so as to improve the network's performance on some task. Back-propagation uses the chain rule from calculus to compute the adjustments to connections that are not on the output edge of the network. Also called 'backprop'.

Bayes' rule. An axiom or basic theorem of probability, that the conditional probability of A given B equals the conditional probability of B given A times the probability of A divided by the probability of B: $P(A|B) = P(B|A) \ P(A)/P(B)$.

Brainstem. The lowest part of the brain, consisting of the midbrain, pons, and medulla, which runs into the spinal cord.

Cerebellum. A part of the brain involved in controlling bodily motion and in sensorimotor learning.

Cerebrum. The largest part of the brain in humans, consisting of the two wrinkled cerebral hemispheres.

Climbing fibers. One of the two main types of nerve fiber that carry signals to the cerebellum (the other being the mossy fibers). Each climbing fiber winds around the cerebellar Purkinje cells like a climbing vine on a tree.

Cochlea. The spiral cavity in the inner ear where sound waves are converted into neural activity.

Complexity. On analysis, this intuitive concept resolves into a number of distinct, technical notions, including algorithmic information content, logical depth and crypticity.

Cortex. The outer layer of the cerebrum or cerebellum, composed of folded gray matter.

Crypticity. A measure of complexity, in a sense the reverse of logical depth. It quantifies how difficult it is to deduce, based on examination of a pattern, the simplest computer program that would generate it.

Degrees of freedom. A system has n degrees of freedom, or equivalently n dimensions, if, roughly speaking, it can be described with n numbers; that is, each distinct state of the system can be labeled uniquely with a set of n numbers.

Derivative. Mathematical term for rate of change. For instance, a derivative can quantify how the position of a car is changing as a function of time, or how the height of the land is changing as a function of longitude. The name derivative is unfortunate because it conveys nothing of the meaning. Isaac Newton, one of the people who discovered derivatives, called them 'fluxions', which is much better.

Differentiator. Mathematical operator that computes derivatives, or in other words rates of change. Its output is the rate of change of its input.

Dimension. A system is n-dimensional if it has n degrees of freedom; that is, roughly speaking, it can be described with n numbers.

Donders' law. States that the eye always adopts the same torsional angle (or angle of twist about its own line of sight) every time it looks in any given direction. Donders' law holds fairly exactly when you keep your head still and look around at distant objects. More generally, a system is said to obey Donders' law if one or more of its potential degrees of freedom are not allowed to vary independently, but are constrained to be some function of the other degrees of freedom.

Energy landscape. Of a neural network: a graph of performance versus synaptic settings. Though normally very high-dimensional, the graph is usefully pictured as a surface in three-dimensional space. All the graph's axes but one represent the strengths of the synapses in the network; these axes span synaptic space, and are pictured as a horizontal plane. The one remaining axis, pictured as vertical, represents the network's error or success on some task. That error or success varies depending on the synaptic strengths, so the energy landscape is higher over some portions of synaptic space than over others.

Filter. Usually in mathematics (and always in this book) an operator that transforms temporal patterns. A high-pass filter passes on rapidly fluctuating signals and filters out steady or slowly oscillating ones. A low-pass filter passes on steady or slowly oscillating signals and filters out rapidly fluctuating ones.

Fovea. The small disk at the center of the retina, specialized for high-acuity vision. In humans it is 5 degrees across, or about as wide as three fingers viewed at the end of your outstretched arm.

Graduated non-convexity. A technique for finding the global optimum, or lowest point, of a complex energy landscape. The method is to approximate the landscape with a simpler one, find the global optimum for that simple case, and then repeat the procedure with gradually more complicated surfaces that are closer and closer matches to the one of interest.

Information. As defined by Shannon, the amount of information in an event, in bits, is the number of yes-or-no questions you would need to ask, and have answered correctly, on average, to deduce which event, from some specified set of possibilities, had happened.

Integrator. Mathematical term for an operator that computes a running sum of its inputs, like a car odometer computing mileage by counting up axle rotations.

Confusingly, the word 'integrate' is often used in neuroscience, as in daily life (but not in this book), to mean 'bring together' or 'orchestrate'. A better name for the mathematical concept might have been 'accumulator'.

Inverse. The inverse of an operator undoes it, so if you hook up an operator and its inverse in series and put a signal through both it will emerge unchanged. Many operators in technology and in biological sensors, brains, and muscles have no inverses, meaning they can't be undone. For instance the operation of squaring is not invertible, because if you know, say, that x^2 is 4, you can't 'desquare' 4 and be sure of getting back x, because you don't know whether x was 2 or –2.

Iteration. A stepwise computation where an operator repeatedly acts on its own previous outputs. Iterative computations can be performed by looping, or recurrent, networks.

Labyrinth. The inner ear, containing the sensors for sound, motion, and gravity.

Linear. In mathematics, a function or transformation is linear if it preserves sums and scaling; that is, L is linear if, for any numbers a and b and any inputs x and y, $L(ax + by) = aL(x) + bL(y)$.

Listing's law. States that the torsional angle of the eye is always zero.

Logical depth. Of a string of 0s and 1s: a measure of complexity; roughly the length of time that a computer of some standardized sort would have to run to generate and print out the string if it were running the simplest program that does so.

Mossy fibers. One of the two main types of fiber (the other being the climbing fibers) that carry signals to the cerebellum. In the cerebellar cortex, mossy fibers contact huge numbers of granule cells, whose axons, called parallel fibers, carry data to Purkinje cells.

Motor neuron. A neuron (nerve cell) that projects to and excites a muscle.

Neural network. A set of mathematical operators that communicate via a web of connections, like neurons in the brain.

Neuron. A nerve cell.

Non-commutativity. An operation is said to be non-commutative when order makes a difference to the outcome. For example, division is non-commutative because 3 divided by 4 does not equal 4 divided by 3. In non-commutative algebra, unlike in normal arithmetic, the operation of multiplication is non-commutative. This sort of algebra is needed to describe rotary motion, so the brain circuits that deal with rotations, for instance of the eyes and joints, must perform non-commutative algebra.

Nucleus. 1. A discrete group of neurons in the brain, 2. The part in most cells of the body that contains (almost all of) the genome.

Nystagmus. Alternating quick and slow rotations of the eye in opposite directions, seen in certain brain disorders and in normal people who are rotating or viewing a moving scene.

Olive. The inferior olivary nucleus in the brainstem is the source of all climbing fibers to the cerebellum.

Optokinesis. Eye movements that track *en bloc* motion of a large portion of the visual field.

Otolith organs. Sensors in the inner ear that measure gravity and the translational acceleration of the head.

Parallel fibers. The main source of sensory, cognitive, and motor data to the Purkinje cells of the cerebellum.

Proprioception. The sense of body position, derived from sensors in the muscles, tendons, and joints.

Purkinje cells. The sole output cells of the computational network of 70 billion neurons in the cerebellar cortex.

Pursuit. The smooth eye rotations we use to track small moving objects. Also called 'smooth pursuit'.

Recurrent network. A neural network with loops.

Retina. The sheet of light-sensitive cells lining most of the inside of the eyeball.

Rotation. Motion that changes the orientation of a thing, as opposed to translation, which changes the location.

Saccade. A quick eye movement, usually used to redirect the line of sight to a new object of interest, though saccades can also twist the eye about its line of sight.

Semicircular canals. Sensors in the inner ear that measure head rotation.

Somaphone. An instrument for listening to the heart, lungs, abdomen, and vasculature throughout the body (from Greek *soma* 'body' and *phone* 'sound').

Synapse. A connection between neurons, through which they communicate.

Synaptic space. Mathematical space where each point represents a set of values for the synapses in a neural network. Synaptic space is the 'floor' or 'ground plane' of the energy landscape for learning

Translation. Motion that changes the location of a thing, as opposed to rotation, which changes the orientation.

Vector. An entity with length and direction. You can picture a vector as an arrow, though vectors can exist in mathematical spaces with unpicturably many dimensions. You can also represent a vector by an ordered set of numbers, called coordinates, which give the extent of the vector in different dimensions; for instance, 3 m forward, 2 m left, 1 m up.

Vestibulo-ocular reflex (VOR). A relatively simple sensorimotor system that helps stabilize the eyeball in space. It measures head motion using sensors in and adjacent to the vestibulum, a chamber in the labyrinth (the inner ear), and conveys signals to the eye muscles to counterrotate the eyes.

Notes and references

1. Brodal, A., *Neurological Anatomy in Relation to Clinical Medicine*. 1981, Oxford: Oxford University Press.
2. Parent, A., *Carpenter's Human Neuroanatomy*. 9th edn, 1996, Media, PA: Williams and Wilkins.
3. That natural selection built our brains doesn't of course mean that it is the sole source of all the order in them. Clearly the laws of physics and the initial state of the universe contributed as well, because they determined what materials selection had to work with, and for that matter they gave rise to natural selection itself. But natural selection is the reason our brains are so well designed, compared to the enormous range of other, possible brains that are also compatible with the laws of physics but are far less capable than ours.
4. Theme song for 'The Beverly Hillbillies'.
5. Turing, A.M., Computing machinery and intelligence. *Mind*, 1950, **59**(236), 433–460.
6. Pinker, S., *How the Mind Works*. 1997, New York: W. W. Norton and Company.
7. Dawkins, R., *The Extended Phenotype: The Long Reach of the Gene*. 2nd edn, 1999, Oxford: Oxford University Press.
8. Gould, S.J., *Ever Since Darwin*. 1991, London: Penguin Books.
9. There are several variants of the golem legend, some pre-dating the real Rabbi Judah Loewe, who lived from 1525 to 1609. People have speculated that those versions where the creature runs amok may have inspired Mary Shelley to write *Frankenstein*. The golem story appealed to Norbert Wiener, the inventor of cybernetics, because of the creature's computer-like way of doing exactly what it was ordered to do rather than what it was supposed to do.
10. Waugh, E., *Brideshead Revisited*. 1962, London: Penguin Books.
11. Banville, J., *Dr Copernicus*. 1976, London: Random House.
12. Hofstadter, D.R., *Goedel, Escher, Bach: an Eternal Golden Braid*. 1979, New York: Basic Books.
13. Penrose, R., *The Emperor's New Mind*. 1989, Oxford: Oxford University Press.
14. An analog computer is not a Turing machine because its currents are not restricted to a finite set of discrete levels, but slide smoothly among an infinity of values. If electric currents are not really continuous but quantized, an analog computer may be a Turing machine after all.
15. Blasdel, G.G., Orientation selectivity, preference and continuity in monkey striate cortex. *Journal of Neuroscience*, 1992, **12**(8), 3139–3161.
16. Howard, I.P. and B.J. Rogers, *Binocular Vision and Stereopsis*, Oxford Psychology Series no 29. 1995, New York: Oxford University Press.
17. Robinson, A., *Non-standard Analysis*. 1996, Princeton, NJ: Princeton University Press.

18. Chaitin, G.J., A theory of program size formally identical to information theory. *Journal of the Association for Computing Machinery*, 1975, **22**(3), 329–340

19. Gell-Mann, M., *The Quark and the Jaguar*. 1994, New York: W. H. Freeman.

20. Estimates vary, but the prevailing view seems to be that the brain contains 100 billion neurons, considerably more glial cells, and between 100 trillion and a quadrillion synapses.

21. Each base pair may contain somewhat less than 2 bits of information. Triplets of bases, called codons, code amino acids, plus a small number of stop signals which terminate protein strings. As there are only 20 different amino acids in the human body, each codon carries only about log 20 bits of information, plus a little for the stop markers, in any case fewer than 5 bits, which means less than 1.7 bits per base. On the other hand, maybe the different codons for a single amino acid do have subtly different chemical effects on DNA behavior, so it may be safer to stick with the 2 bit estimate.

22. Venter, J.C., *et al.*, (*Science*, 2001, 291: 1304–1351) estimate that just 1.1 to 1.4 per cent of the genome is transcribed to make proteins. Some of the rest regulates transcription, but most of it is widely believed to have no function—it accumulated over the eons and was never weeded out because it doesn't do much harm, or at least, it is believed to have no very specific role which would depend on its precise sequence of base pairs.

23. Dyson, F., *Origins of Life*. 1999, Cambridge: Cambridge University Press.

24. Kauffman, S.A., *The Origins of Order: Self-Organization and Selection in Evolution*. 1993, Oxford: Oxford University Press.

25. Maynard Smith, J. and E. Szathmáry, *The Origins of Life*. 1999, Oxford: Oxford University Press.

26. Cairns-Smith, A.G., *Seven Clues to the Origin of Life: a Scientific Detective Story*. 1991, Cambridge: Cambridge University Press.

27. Bennett, C.H., Logical depth and physical complexity. In *The Universal Turing Machine: a Half-Century Survey*, ed. R. Herkin. 1988, Oxford: Oxford University Press, pp. 227–257.

28. Bennett, C.H., Dissipation, information, computational complexity and the definition of organization. In *Emerging Syntheses in Science*, ed. D. Pines. 1988, Reading, MA: Addison-Wesley, pp. 215–233.

29. Bennett, C.H., How to define complexity in physics, and why. In *Complexity, Entropy and the Physics of Information*, ed. W. Zurek. 1990, Reading, MA: Addison-Wesley, pp. 137–148.

30. Hebb, D.O., *The Organization of Behavior: a Neuropsychological Theory*. 1949, New York: Wiley.

31. Martin, T.A., *et al.*, Throwing while looking through prisms. II. Specificity and storage of multiple gaze-throw calibrations. *Brain*, 1996, **119**(4), 1199–1211.

32. C., J., Living without a balancing mechanism. *New England Journal of Medicine*, 1952, **246**, 458–460.

33. Carl, J.R. and R.S. Gellman, Human smooth pursuit: stimulus-dependent responses. *Journal of Neurophysiology*, 1987, **57**, 1446–1463.

34. Viirre, E., *et al.*, A reexamination of the gain of the vestibuloocular reflex. *Journal of Neurophysiology*, 1986, **56**(2), 439–450.

35. Lorente de Nó, R., Vestibulo-ocular reflex arc. *Archives of Neurology and Psychiatry*, 1933, **30**, 245–291.

36. Szentágothai, J., The elementary vestibulo-ocular reflex arc. *Journal of Neurophysiology*, 1950, **13**, 395–407.
37. Smith, P.F. and I.S. Curthoys, Mechanisms of recovery following unilateral labyrinthectomy: a review. *Brain Research Reviews*, 1989, **14**, 155–180.
38. Zee, D.S., T.J. Preziosi, and L.R. Proctor, Bechterew's phenomenon in a human patient. *Annals of Neurology*, 1982, **12**, 495–496.
39. Katsarkas, A., H.L. Galiana, Bechterew's phenomenon in humans. *Acta Oto-Laryngologica Supplement (Stockholm)*, 1984, **406**, 95–100.
40. Istl-Lenz, Y., D. Hyden, and D.W.F. Schwartz, Response of the human vestibulo-ocular reflex following long-term 2× magnified visual input. *Experimental Brain Research*, 1985, **57**, 448–455.
41. Gonshor, A. and G. Melvill Jones, Extreme vestibulo-ocular adaptation induced by prolonged optical reversal of vision. *Journal of Physiology (London)*, 1976. **256**, 381–414.
42. Khater, T.T., J.F. Baker, and B.W. Peterson, Dynamics of adaptive change in human vestibulo-ocular reflex direction. *Journal of Vestibular Research*, 1990, **1**, 23–29.
43. Obviously, if you want to perform several different linear operations you need several linear neurons, so in that sense multiple linear cells can do things no single cell can.
44. Ripley, B.D., *Pattern Recognition and Neural Networks*. 1996, Cambridge: Cambridge University Press.
45. Rumelhart, D.E. and J.L. McClelland, *Parallel Distributed Processing: Explorations in the Microstructure of Cognition*. 1986, Cambridge, MA: MIT Press.
46. Hinton, G.E., How neural networks learn from experience. *Scientific American*, 1992, **267**(3), 105–109.
47. Werbos, P.J., The cytoskeleton: why it may be crucial to human learning and to neurocontrol. *Nanobiology*, 1992, **1**, 75–95.
48. Tao, H.W. and M. Poo, Retrograde signaling at central synapses. *Proceedings of the National Academy of Sciences of the USA*, 2001, **98**(20), 11009–11015.
49. Poo, M.M., Neurotrophins as synaptic modulators. *Nature Reviews Neuroscience*, 2001, **2**(1), 24–32.
50. Stork, D., Is backpropagation biologically plausible? 1989 *IEEE INNS International Joint Conference on Neural Networks*, 1989, San Diego: IEEE TAB Neural Network Committee, 241–246.
51. Fitzsimonds, R.M., H.J. Song, and M.M. Poo, Propagation of activity-dependent synaptic depression in simple neural networks. *Nature*, 1997, **388**, 439–448.
52. Tao, H.W., *et al.*, Selective presynaptic propagation of long-term potentiation in defined neural networks. *Journal of Neuroscience*, 2000, **20**(9), 3233–3243.
53. Geman, S., E. Bienenstock, and R. Doursat, Neural networks and the bias/variance dilemma. *Neural Computation*, 1992, **4**, 1–58.
54. Press, W.H., *et al.*, *Numerical Recipes in C*. 2nd edn, 1992, Cambridge: Cambridge University Press. This book doesn't discuss brain simulations specifically, but it deals with the underlying issues of optimization and dynamics.
55. Kirkpatrick, S., C.D. Gelatt, and M.P. Vecchi, Optimization by simulated annealing. *Science*, 1983, **220**, 671–680.
56. Blake, A. and A. Zisserman, *Visual Reconstruction*. 1987, Cambridge, MA: MIT Press.
57. Holland, J., *Adaptation in Natural and Artificial Systems*. 1975, Ann Arbor, MI: University of Michigan Press.

58. Levy, S., *Artificial Life.* 1993, London: Penguin.
59. Waldrop, M.M., *Complexity: the Emerging Science at the Edge of Order and Chaos.* 1992, New York: Simon and Schuster.
60. Mel, B.W., *Connectionist Robot Motion Planning.* 1990, Cambridge, MA: Academic Press.
61. Saarinen, J. and T. Kohonen, Self-organized formation of colour maps in a model cortex. *Perception,* 1985, **14**(6), 711–719.
62. Lange, W., Cell number and cell density in the cerebellar cortex of man and other mammals. *Cell Tissue Research,* 1975, **157**, 115–124.
63. Lisberger, S.G., F.A. Miles, and D.S. Zee, Signals used to compute errors in the monkey vestibuloocular reflex: possible role of the flocculus. *Journal of Neurophysiology,* 1984, **52**, 1140–1153.
64. Optican, L.M., D.S. Zee, and F.A. Miles, Floccular lesions abolish adaptive control of post-saccadic drift in primates. *Experimental Brain Research,* 1986, **64**, 596–598.
65. Takagi, M., D.S. Zee, and R.J. Tamargo, Effects of lesions of the oculomotor vermis on eye movements in primate: saccades. *Journal of Neurophysiology,* 1998, **80**, 1911–1930.
66. Marr, D., A theory of cerebellar cortex. *Journal of Physiology,* 1969, **202**(2), 437–470.
67. Albus, J., A theory of cerebellar function. *Mathematical Biosciences,* 1971, **10**, 25–61.
68. Ekerot, C.F. and M. Kano, Long-term depression of parallel fibre synapses following stimulation of climbing fibres. *Brain Research,* 1985, **342**(2), 357–360.
69. Ito, M., Long-term depression as a memory process in the cerebellum. *Neuroscience Research,* 1986, **3**(6), 531–539.
70. Robinson, D.A. and L.M. Optican, Adaptive plasticity in the oculomotor system. In *Lesion Induced Neuronal Plasticity in Sensorimotor Systems,* ed. H. Floir and W. Precht. 1981, Berlin: Springer, pp. 295–304.
71. Highstein, S.M., Role of the flocculus of the cerebellum in motor learning of the vestibulo-ocular reflex. *Otolaryngology—Head and Neck Surgery,* 1998, **119**(3), 212–220.
72. Ito, M., Synaptic plasticity in the cerebellar cortex and its role in motor learning. *Canadian Journal of Neurological Sciences,* 1993, **20**(Supplement 3), S70–S74.
73. Haddad, G.M., J.L. Demer, and D.A. Robinson, The effect of lesions of the dorsal cap of the inferior olive on the vestibulo-ocular and optokinetic systems of the cat. *Brain Research,* 1980, **185**, 265–276.
74. Campbell, N.C., *et al.,* Interaction between mossy fibre and climbing fibre responses in Purkinje cells. *Acta Morphologica Hungarica,* 1983, **31**(1–3), 181–192.
75. Lisberger, S.G., Physiologic basis for motor learning in the vestibulo-ocular reflex. *Otolaryngology—Head and Neck Surgery,* 1998, **119**(1), 43–48.
76. Baldwin, J.M., A new factor in evolution. *The American Naturalist,* 1896, **30**, 441–451, 536–553.
77. Hinton, G.E. and S.J. Nowlan, How learning can guide evolution. *Complex Systems,* 1987, **1**, 495–502.

78. Actually, keeping your eye velocity equal to -1 times your head velocity will stabilize your retinal images reasonably well only if you are spinning in one spot and everything you can see is at least a meter or so away from your face. As I discuss in Chapter 9, the task of keeping your images stationary under other conditions is more complex.

79. Lopez-Barneo, J., et al., Neuronal activity in prepositus nucleus correlated with eye movement in the alert cat. Journal of Neurophysiology, 1982, **47**, 329-352.

80. McFarland, J.L. and A.F. Fuchs, Discharge patterns in nucleus prepositus hypoglossi and adjacent medial vestibular nucleus during horizontal eye movement in behaving macaques. Journal of Neurophysiology, 1992, **68**, 319-332.

81. Crawford, J.D., W. Cadera, and T. Vilis, Generation of torsional and vertical eye position signals by the interstitial nucleus of Cajal. Science, 1991, **252**(5012), 1551-1553.

82. Cannon, S.C. and D.A. Robinson, Loss of the neural integrator of the oculomotor system from brain stem lesions in monkey. Journal of Neurophysiology, 1987, **57**, 1383-1409.

83. Cheron, G. and E. Godaux, Disabling of the oculomotor neural integrator by kainic acid injections in the prepositus-vestibular complex of the cat. Journal of Physiology (London), 1987, **394**, 267-290.

84. Carpenter, R.H.S., Cerebellectomy and the transfer function of the vestibulo-ocular reflex in the decerebrate cat. Proceedings of the Royal Society of London Series B: Biological Sciences, 1972, **181**, 353-374.

85. Raphan, T., V. Matsuo, and B. Cohen, Velocity storage in the vestibulo-ocular reflex arc (VOR). Experimental Brain Research, 1979, **35**, 229-248. In monkeys the canals respond for about 20 s; in humans the duration is thought to be similar.

86. Pinna, B. and G.J. Brelstaff, A new visual illusion of relative motion. Vision Research, 2000, **40**, 2091-2096. Other renderings of this illusion, much more impressive than mine, can be found on the Internet; when I first saw them, I thought the computer was monitoring my head motion and altering the screen image. Pinna and Brelstaff attribute the illusion to misjudged motions of image elements called polarities.

87. Marr, D., Vision. 1982, New York: W. H. Freeman and Company.

88. Schweigart, G., T. Mergner, and G. Barnes, Eye movements during combined pursuit, optokinetic and vestibular stimulation in macaque monkey. Experimental Brain Research, 1999, **127**, 54-66.

89. Cannon, S.C., D.A. Robinson, and S. Shamma, A proposed neural network for the integrator of the oculomotor system. Biological Cybernetics, 1983, **49**, 127-136.

90. Cannon, S.C. and D.A. Robinson, An improved neural-network model for the neural integrator of the oculomotor system: more realistic neuron behavior. Biological Cybernetics, 1985, **53**, 93-108.

91. Kramer, P.D., M. Shelhamer, and D.S. Zee, Short-term adaptation of the phase of the vestibulo-ocular reflex (VOR) in normal human subjects. Experimental Brain Research, 1995, **106**(2), 318-326.

92. Collins, W.E., Special effects of brief periods of visual fixation on nystagmus and sensations of turning. Aerospace Medicine, 1968, **39**, 257-266.

93. Collins, W.E., Habituation of vestibular responses with and without visual stimulation. In *Handbook of Sensory Physiology*, volume VI(2), ed. H.H Kornhuber. 1974, Berlin: Springer, pp. 369–388.

94. Bi, G.Q. and M.M. Poo, Synaptic modification by correlated activity: Hebb's postulate revisited. *Annual Review of Neuroscience*, 2001, **24**, 139–166.

95. Pineda, F.J., Dynamics and architecture for neural computation. *Journal of Complexity*, 1988, **4**, 216–245.

96. Anastasio, T.J., Simulating vestibular compensation using recurrent back-propagation. *Biological Cybernetics*, 1992, **66**(5), 389–397.

97. Arnold, D.B. and D.A. Robinson, The oculomotor integrator: testing of a neural network model. *Experimental Brain Research*, 1997, **113**(1), 57–74.

98. I got this number from a TV commercial, and I recall reading something similar in my *How and Why Wonder Book of the Human Body*. Most anatomy texts are evasive about the exact number of skeletal muscles in the body, presumably because it is not always clear whether a branching bundle of muscle tissue should be regarded as one muscle or several.

99. Huxley, H.E. and J. Hanson, Changes in the cross striations of muscle during contraction and stretch and their structural interpretation. *Nature*, 1954, **173**, 973–976.

100. Huxley, A.F., Review lecture: Muscular contraction. *Journal of Physiology*, 1974, **243**, 1–43.

101. Zajac, F.E., Muscle and tendon: properties, models, scaling, and application to biomechanics and motor control. *CRC Critical Reviews in Biomedical Engineering*, 1989, **17**(4), 359–411.

102. The product of a muscle's force and velocity is called its power output, and it is positive when the force and the velocity have the same direction. This happens only when the muscle is contracting; a stretching muscle may exert a lot of force but it does no work and puts out no power. Power output peaks when a muscle contracts at about 30 per cent of its maximum shortening velocity. When bicycling, you change gears to keep your muscle velocity near the maximum-power point.

103. Actually, Newton said that force equals the rate of change of momentum. As momentum is mass times velocity, its rate of change equals mass times acceleration if the mass of the moving object is constant; this is not the case for, say, a spacecraft that is rapidly burning off tons of fuel and shedding booster rockets, but it is true enough for the motile parts of the human body.

104. Robinson, D.A., Oculomotor unit behavior in the monkey. *Journal of Neurophysiology*, 1970, **33**(3), 393–404.

105. Leigh, R.J. and D.S. Zee, *The Neurology of Eye Movements*, 3rd edn. 1999, New York: Oxford University Press.

106. The pattern isn't a precise pulse-step, probably because it is hard to create abrupt force changes with muscle, and because moving the eye isn't precisely equivalent to moving springs in glue.

107. Collins, C.C., The human oculomotor control system. In *Basic Mechanisms of Ocular Motility and their Clinical Implications*, ed. G. Lennerstrand and P. Bach-y-Rita. 1975, Oxford: Pergamon, pp. 145–180.

108. Robinson, D.A., Oculomotor control signals. In *Basic Mechanisms of Ocular Motility and their Clinical Implications.*, ed. G. Lennerstrand and P. Bach-y-Rita. 1975, Oxford: Pergamon, pp. 337–374.

109. Van Gisbergen, J.A.M., D.A. Robinson, and S.A. Gielen, A quantitative analysis of generation of saccadic eye movements by burst neurons. *Journal of Neurophysiology*, 1981, **45**, 417–442.

110. Partridge, L.D., Modifications of neural output signals by muscles: a frequency response study. *Journal of Applied Physiology*, 1965, **20**, 150–156.

111. Burke, R.E., P. Rudomin, and F.E. Zajac, The effect of activation history on tension production by individual muscle units. *Brain Research*, 1976, **109**, 515–529.

112. There are many steps between neural firing and force production, and the dynamics are complex, but a low-pass filter is a useful approximation.

113. Hallett, M., B.T. Shahani, and R.R. Young, EMG analysis of stereotyped voluntary movements in man. *Journal of Neurology Neurosurgery and Psychiatry*, 1975, **38**(12), 1154–1162.

114. Hannaford, B. and L. Stark, Roles of the elements of the triphasic control signal. *Experimental Neurology*, 1985, **90**(3), 619–634.

115. Lan, N., Analysis of an optimal control model of multi-joint arm movements. *Biological Cybernetics*, 1997, **76**(2), 107–117.

116. Several theorists have observed that the brain, when it moves the arm, seems to be optimizing some variable related to the third derivative of arm position, or jerk. One explanation is that because the equation relating innervation to arm motion is third-order, neural activity is related to jerk, so by minimizing jerk-related variables the brain may actually be minimizing its own activity, maybe to save metabolic fuel or to reduce noise.

117. Tijssen, M.A., *et al.*, Optokinetic afternystagmus in humans: normal values of amplitude, time constant, and asymmetry. *Annals of Otology Rhinology and Laryngology*, 1989, **98**(9), 741–746.

118. Segal, B.N. and S. Liben, Modulation of human velocity storage sampled during intermittently-illuminated optokinetic stimulation. *Experimental Brain Research*, 1985, **59**(3), 515–523.

119. Demer, J.L., S.Y. Oh, and V. Poukens, Evidence for active control of rectus extraocular muscle pulleys. *Investigative Ophthalmology and Visual Science*, 2000, **41**(6), 1280–1290.

120. Demer, J.L., *et al.*, Evidence for fibromuscular pulleys of the recti extraocular muscles. *Investigative Ophthalmology and Visual Science*, 1995, **36**, 1125–1136.

121. I am thinking of mounting a drive to have the muscle pulleys renamed grommets. I have some experience with this sort of thing, having campaigned in medical school to rename the stethoscope. The usual name means a device for looking at the chest, but in fact stethoscopes are used to listen to, not view, many different body parts. I proposed the name 'somaphone'. To its discredit, the medical community ignored me, but maybe neuroscientists will learn from that mistake. It is ironic that Doctors Without Borders, which started a few years earlier, went on to win the Nobel Peace Prize, while my initiative foundered.

122. Optican, L.M. and C. Quaia, Effects of orbital pulleys on the control of eye rotations. In *Vision and Action*, ed. L.R. Harris and M. Jenkins, 1998, New York: Cambridge University Press, pp. 120–138.

123. Quaia, C. and L.M. Optican, Commutative saccadic generator is sufficient to control a 3-D ocular plant with pulleys. *Journal of Neurophysiology*, 1998, **79**(6), 3197–3215.

124. Raphan, T., Modeling control of eye orientation in three dimensions. I. Role of muscle pulleys in determining saccade trajectory. *Journal of Neurophysiology*, 1998, **79**, 2653-2667.

125. Tweed, D., H. Misslisch, and M. Fetter, Testing models of the oculomotor velocity-to-position transformation. *Journal of Neurophysiology*, 1994, **72**(3), 1425-1429.

126. Tweed, D., Kinematic principles of three-dimensional gaze control. In *Three-Dimensional Kinematics of Eye, Head and Limb Movements*, ed. M. Fetter, *et al.* 1997, Amsterdam: Harwood, pp. 17-32.

127. Wiener, N., *Cybernetics: or Control and Communication in the Animal and the Machine*. 1948, Cambridge, MA: MIT Press.

128. Vasari, G., *The Lives of the Artists*. 1998, Oxford: Oxford University Press.

129. Davies, R., *What's Bred in the Bone*. 1985, New York: Viking.

130. Clouzot, H.-G., *Le Mystère Picasso*. 1956.

131. Braak, J.W.G.t., Untersuchungen über optokinetischen Nystagmus. *Archives Néerlandaises de physiologie de l'homme et des animaux* 1936, **21**, 309-376.

132. Mittelstaedt, H., Telotaxis und Optomotorik von Eristalis bei Augeninversion. *Naturwissenschaften*, 1949, **36**, 90-91.

133. When the fly's head is twisted back to its usual posture, the animal's behavior also returns to normal.

134. Stark, L., G. Vossius, and L.R. Young. Predictive control of eye tracking movements. *IRE Transactions on Human Factors in Electronics*, 1962, **HFE-3**, 52-57.

135. Barnes, G.R. and P.T. Asselman, The mechanism of prediction in human smooth pursuit eye movements. *Journal of Physiology (London)*, 1991, **439**, 439-461.

136. Steinbach, M.J., Pursuing the perceptual rather than the retinal stimulus. *Vision Research*, 1976, **16**(12), 1371-1376.

137. Gregory, R.L., Eye movements and the stability of the visual world. *Nature*, 1958, **192**, 1214-1216.

138. Jordan, S., Ocular pursuit movement as a function of visual and proprioceptive stimulation. *Vision Research*, 1970, **10**, 775-780.

139. Gauthier, G.M. and J.M. Hofferer, Eye tracking of self-moved targets in the absence of vision. *Experimental Brain Research*, 1976, **26**(2), 121-139.

140. Lackner, J.R., Some proprioceptive influences on the perceptual representation of body shape and orientation. *Brain*, 1988, **111**, 281-297.

141. Guthrie, B., J.D.Porter and D.L. Sparks, Corollary discharge provides accurate eye position information to the oculomotor system *Science*, 1983, 221, 1193-1195.

142. Zee, D., *et al.*, Slow saccades in spinocerebellar degeneration. *Archives of Neurology*, 1976, **33**(4), 243-251.

143. Becker, W., *et al.*, Accuracy of goal-directed saccades and mechanisms of error correction. In *Progress in Oculomotor Research*, ed. A.F. Fuchs and W. Becker, 1981, New York: Elsevier, pp. 29-37.

144. Brown, M.A. and P.W. Glimcher, The saccadic system compensates for trajectory perturbations induced by intra-saccadic microstimulation of medium-lead burst neurons. *Abstracts of the Neural Control of Movement Society Meeting*, 2000 (www-ncm.cs.umass.edu/abstracts/2000/238400.html).

145. Optican, L.M. and C. Quaia, Distributed model of collicular and cerebellar function during saccades. *Annals of the New York Academy of Science*, 2002, **956**, 164–177.

146. Abbott, E.A., *Flatland, a Romance of Many Dimensions*. 1976, New York: Buccaneer Books.

147. Strictly speaking, this definition of 'dimension' doesn't quite work, as Georg Cantor showed in the nineteenth century. For a rigorous definition, we have to insist that the n numbers provide a continuous representation, in the mathematical sense. But all the examples in this book are continuous.

148. Chaudhari, N., A.M. Landin, and S.D. Roper, A metabotropic glutamate receptor variant functions as a taste receptor. *Nature Neuroscience*, 2000, **3**(2), 113–119.

149. Hoon, M.A., *et al.*, Putative mammalian taste receptors: a class of taste-specific GPCRs with distinct topographic selectivity. *Cell*, 1999, **96**(4), 541–551.

150. Nelson, G., *et al.*, An amino-acid taste receptor. *Nature*, 2002, **416**(6877), 199–202.

151. In a space of n dimensions, translation has n degrees of freedom, but the number of degrees of freedom of rotation is n-choose-2, which is the number of pairs of items you can choose from a set of n. The reason is that every dimension of rotation corresponds to some plane of rotation. You need two lines to specify a plane, so in an n-dimensional space, where you can find n lines all orthogonal to one another, you can get n-choose-2 planes all orthogonal to one another. The number n-choose-2 grows rapidly as n increases, so the possibilities for rotation quickly outstrip those for translation.

152. Collewijn, H., *et al.*, Human ocular counterroll: assessment of static and dynamic properties from electromagnetic scleral coil recordings. *Experimental Brain Research*, 1985, **59**, 185–196.

153. Merton, P.A., Compensatory rolling movements of the eye. *Journal of Physiology*, 1956, **132**, 25P–27P.

154. Williams, G.C., *Plan and Purpose in Nature*. 1996, London: Weidenfeld and Nicolson.

155. We could rotate the eye three-dimensionally using just *four* muscles, with an arrangements anologous to the one in Fig. 9.1, but our six-muscle design makes more efficient use of force.

156. Tweed, D.B., *et al.*, Non-commutativity in the brain. *Nature*, 1999, **399**(6733), 261–263.

157. No one knows where the VOR's non-commutative operators are located. Some authors have suggested that they are all in the cerebral cortex and that the VOR circuitry in the brainstem is purely commutative. This seems to me unlikely. As far as I can tell, the only motivation for positing a commutative brainstem is a distaste for unorthodox math.

158. Donders, F.C., Beitrag zur Lehre von den Bewegungen des menschlichen Auges. *Hollaendische Beitraege zu den anatomischen und physiologischen Wissenschaften*, Vol. 1. 1848, pp. 105–145.

159. Tweed, D. and T. Vilis, Listing's law for gaze-directing head movements. In *The Head-Neck Sensory-Motor System*, ed. A. Berthoz, W. Graf, and P.P. Vidal. 1992, New York: Oxford University Press, pp. 387–391.

160. Helmholtz, H.v. (and J.P.C. Southall), *Helmholtz's Treatise on Physiological Optics*, 3 Vols., translated from the 3rd German edn, ed. J.P.C. Southall. 1962, New York: Dover Publications.

161. Geometrically it would be possible to obey Listing's law and nevertheless violate Donders' if you could rotate your eye 180 degrees away from primary position, but so far as I am aware no animal exploits this possibility.

162. Sándor, P.S., M.A. Frens, and V. Henn, Chameleon eye position obeys Listing's law. *Vision Research*, 2001, **41**(17), 2245-2251.

163. Hermann von Helmholtz and his arch rival Ewald Hering presented theories about the role of Listing's law. Hering observed that it keeps the retinal images of radial lines 'self-congruent'. That is, if your eye begins in the primary position, looking at the center of a starburst pattern of radiating lines, then as you move your gaze point outward along any one of the lines the retinal image of that line will continue to fall along the same set of receptors as long as your eye rotation obeys Listing's law. It will also continue to excite the same set of orientation detectors in primary visual cortex. Hering didn't know about cortical line detectors, but he did feel that the steady retinal image might make it easier for the brain to identify and locate lines in space. Helmholtz's theory was more involved, but it also maintained that Listing's law optimizes a property of retinal image flow. A century and a half later, it seems clear that both theories are wrong. Retinal image flow depends on the eye's motion with respect to space, so both Helmholtz's and Hering's hypotheses assume that the eye rotates relative to space in the way dictated by Listing's law. We now know that this is not so. The eye rotates relative to the head in accordance with the law, but the head itself also moves during most large gaze shifts, so the overall motion of the eye in space deviates markedly from Listing's law. Therefore it seems unlikely that Listing's law evolved to simplify retinal image flow. Helmholtz and Hering's theories failed because they were too low-dimensional: they neglected relevant degrees of freedom. The theories made sense for an eye rotating in space with three degrees of freedom, but not for an eye rotating in a mobile head, where the two parts together have six degrees of freedom.

164. Fick, A., Die Bewegungen des menschlichen Augapfels. *Zeitschrift für rationelle Medicin*, 1854, **4**, 101-128.

165. Wundt, W., Über die Bewegung der Augen. *Archiv für Ophthalmologie*, 1862, **8**(2), 1-87.

166. Pelisson, D., C. Prablanc, and C. Urquizar, Vestibuloocular reflex inhibition and gaze saccade control characteristics during eye-head orientation in humans. *Journal of Neurophysiology*, 1988, **59**(3), 997-1013.

167. Phillips, J.O., *et al.*, Rapid horizontal gaze movement in the monkey. *Journal of Neurophysiology*, 1995, **73**(4), 1632-1652.

168. Laurutis, V.P. and D.A. Robinson, The vestibulo-ocular reflex during human saccadic eye movements. *Journal of Physiology*, 1986, **373**, 209-233.

169. Guitton, D. and M. Volle, Gaze control in humans: eye-head coordination during orienting movements to targets within and beyond the oculomotor range. *Journal of Neurophysiology*, 1987, **58**(3), 427-459.

170. Tomlinson, R.D. and P.S. Bahra, Combined eye-head gaze shifts in the primate. II. Interactions between saccades and the vestibuloocular reflex. *Journal of Neurophysiology*, 1986, **56**(6), 1558-1570.

171. Tweed, D., T. Haslwanter, and M. Fetter, Optimizing gaze control in three dimensions. *Science*, 1998, **281**(5381), 1363-1366.

172. Head rotation is often described using the three coordinates yaw, pitch, and roll, which originated as nautical terms. Yaw is horizontal rotation about a vertical

axis, as when turning your boat left or right. For landlubbers, an example is the back-and-forth motion used, through much of the Western world, in shaking your head 'no'. Pitch is vertical rotation about a sideways axis, as when the prow of your longship descends as you come over the crest of a wave. An example of head pitch is nodding 'yes'. Roll, a term dating from the Dark Ages when bands of fierce bakers used to sail down from Norway to harry the Frankish coast, refers to an alarming sort of rotation about the long axis of the boat. You are rolling your head when you slap your shoulders with your ears.

173. Paige, G.D., Linear vestibulo-ocular reflex (LVOR) and modulation by vergence. *Acta Oto-Laryngologica Supplement (Stockholm)*, 1991, **481**, 282–286.

174. Blakemore, C. and M. Donaghy, Co-ordination of head and eyes in the gaze changing behaviour of cats. *Journal of Physiology*, 1980, **300**, 317–335.

175. Paige, G.D. and D.L. Tomko, Eye movement responses to linear head motion in the squirrel monkey. I. Basic characteristics. *Journal of Neurophysiology*, 1991, **65**(5), 1170–1182.

176. Paige, G.D. and D.L. Tomko, Eye movement responses to linear head motion in the squirrel monkey. II. Visual-vestibular interactions and kinematic considerations. *Journal of Neurophysiology*, 1991, **65**(5), 1183–1196.

177. Tomko, D.L. and G.D. Paige, Linear vestibuloocular reflex during motion along axes between nasooccipital and interaural. *Annals of the New York Academy of Science*, 1992, **656**, 233–241.

178. Harris, C.M. and D.M. Wolpert, Signal-dependent noise determines motor planning. *Nature*, 1998, **394**(6695), 780–784.

179. Kalman, R.E., A new approach to linear filtering and prediction problems. *Transactions of the ASME—Journal of Basic Engineering (Series D)*, 1960, **82**, 35–45.

180. I don't necessarily mean to sound like some kind of Frequentist here. The point is merely that the brain estimates the relevant probabilities from the frequencies.

181. Anastasio, T.J., P.E. Patton, and K. Belkacem-Boussaid, Using Bayes' rule to model multisensory enhancement in the superior colliculus. *Neural Computation*, 2000, **12**(5), 1165–1187.

182. A similar calculation reveals the location of Tartarus, the pit below Hades in Greek mythology where the Titans are chained. A hammer dropped from the Earth's surface falls for nine days and nights before it reaches Tartarus. Assuming a constant acceleration of 1g, this formula places Tartarus about 2.97 billion kilometers below Greece. In fact the acceleration would not be constant, owing to air resistance and the diminishing force of gravity near the Earth's core, but the mythologists didn't know that.

183. Seidman, S.H., L. Telford, and G.D. Paige, Tilt perception during dynamic linear acceleration. *Experimental Brain Research*, 1998, **119**(3), 307–314.

184. Mayne, R., A systems concept of the vestibular organs. In *Handbook of Sensory Physiology*, volume VI(2), ed. H.H, Kornhuber. 1974, Berlin: Springer, pp. 493–580.

185. Angelaki, D.E., *et al.*, Computation of inertial motion: neural strategies to resolve ambiguous otolith information. *Journal of Neuroscience*, 1999, **19**(1), 316–327.

186. Angelaki, D.E., M. Wei, and D.M. Merfeld, Vestibular discrimination of gravity and translational acceleration. *Annals of the New York Academy of Science*, 2001, **942**, 114–127.

187. Merfeld, D.M., Modeling human vestibular responses during eccentric rotation and off vertical axis rotation. *Acta Oto-Laryngologica Supplement*, 1995, **520**(2), 354–359.

188. Glasauer, S., Interaction of semicircular canals and otoliths in the processing structure of the subjective zenith. *Annals of the New York Academy of Science*, 1992, **656**, 847–849.

189. Jaynes's book is to be published by Cambridge University Press, but is at the moment still available on the Internet at http://omega.albany.edu:8008/JaynesBook.html.

Index